CORDYCEPS

China's Healing Mushroom

GEORGES M. HALPERN, MD, PhD

AVERY PUBLISHING GROUP

Garden City Park • New York

The information and procedures contained in this book are based upon the research and the personal and professional experiences of the author. They are not intended as a substitute for consulting with your physician or other health care provider. The publisher and author are not responsible for any adverse effects or consequences resulting from the use of any of the suggestions, preparations, or procedures discussed in this book. All matters pertaining to your physical health should be supervised by a health care professional.

Cover Design: Phaedra Mastrocola
Typesetter: Gary A. Rosenberg
Editor: Joan Taber Altieri
Printer: Paragon Press, Honesdale, PA

Avery Publishing Group
120 Old Broadway
Garden City Park, NY 11040
1-800-548-5757
www.averypublishing.com

Cataloging-in-Publication Data
Halpern, Georges M.
    Cordyceps : China's healing mushroom/
Georges M. Halpern.—1st ed.
    p. cm.
    Includes bibliographical references and
index.
    ISBN: 0-89529-811-2

    1. Cordyceps—Therapeutic use. 2. Medicine,
Chinese. I. Title.

RM666.M87H35 1999   615'.3295'67
                                     QBI99-152

Printed in the United States of America

10 9 8 7 6 5 4 3

CONTENTS

INTRODUCTION

Cordyceps: China's Healing Mushroom is the first book of its kind. It is dedicated to bringing information about the healing powers of a medicinal mushroom known as cordyceps to Western readers. The wonders of cordyceps have been known in China for at least 1,000 years, where it is recognized as a national medicinal treasure, a precious and virtually sacred tonic. Cordyceps first received world attention when American news reporters interviewed China's record-breaking athletes, who revealed that they routinely took cordyceps as a post-exercise recovery food. Since that time, research on cordyceps has greatly increased. In clinical studies designed to uncover the secret of its health benefits, over 2,000 patients have been treated with cordyceps. More often than not, the results have been excellent.

Cordyceps is among the safest medicinal foods. Research has shown that it may be useful in the treatment of cardiac arrhythmia, angina pectoris, liver diseases, and cancer. These uses help clarify the meaning of an ancient document that praises cordyceps as a powerful tonic capable of restoring health. Researchers now know that cordyceps is beneficial to the heart, liver, kidneys, respiratory tract, and immune system. It is recommended as a general health supplement to increase vitality and energy, and it is prescribed for some very specific ailments, including opium addiction, infertility, sexual dysfunction, chronic coughing and bronchial problems, anemia, emphysema, tuberculosis, and jaundice. The list does not end here. Let's look at the disorders that are most often treated with cordyceps.

- *Heart Disease.* Various forms of heart disease have been treated with cordyceps with good results. In one study, over 84 percent of patients with cardiac arrhythmia improved following treatment with cordyceps. This figure compared with a 10-percent improvement in patients taking a placebo. Patients with chronic heart failure who were given a combination of cordyceps and conventional drugs fared better than those taking conventional medications alone. Significant improvements were found in the cordyceps group in stroke volume, heartbeat, cardiac output, general activity, and mental state.

    Pulmonary heart disease patients have also responded positively to treatment with cordyceps. In one study, over 90 percent of patients who took cordyceps showed improvements in pulmonary function, emotional well-being, heart function, and sleep.

- *Cholesterol.* Clinical studies have shown that cordyceps can reduce the amount of "bad" LDL cholesterol, and increase the amount "good" HDL cholesterol in people of all ages. In one study, cordyceps lowered total cholesterol levels by over 17 percent, and it lowered the cholesterol levels of patients with coronary heart disease by 21 percent.

- *Liver Disease.* Studies have shown that cordyceps can

help treat some liver diseases. In one clinical trial, cirrhosis of the liver following hepatitis was treated with cordyceps, which was found to improve symptoms and liver-cell structures dramatically. In fact, cirrhotic cells disappeared in 70 percent of the patients. In the treatment of hepatitis B, an extract of the plant was reported to have completely changed antibody readings in nearly 40 percent of patients. In cases of chronic hepatitis-B infections, researchers reported that cordyceps helped bring about improvements or complete recovery in a significant number of patients.

- *Sexual Dysfunction in Men.* Cordyceps has an ancient reputation as an effective treatment for male impotence. Its use for this purpose was better known among the royal families and the upper classes who could afford the mushroom, which was once a rare and extremely costly item. In recent times, researchers have demonstrated that cordyceps can benefit many men who have problems involving sexual function.

- *Kidney Problems.* The primary use of cordyceps in traditional Chinese medicine is in the treatment of kidney disorders. Research has confirmed that the mushroom can improve kidney function. And in kidney transplant patients, cordyceps was shown to return levels of infection-fighting T cells to normal. Other research has found fewer signs of kidney toxicity of drugs in transplant patients who take cordyceps. In addition, doctors have discovered that the benefits of cordyceps increase over time—the longer patients take the mushroom, the more their health improves.

- *Respiratory Functions.* A famous adage in traditional Chinese medicine states that cordyceps goes to the "lung channel." In fact, this has been corroborated by clinical studies. A preliminary study found that middle-aged and elderly patients who took cordyceps for chronic obstructive pulmonary disease (COPD) showed notable improvements in their conditions. Coughing, gasping for air, and general physical signs of COPD were alleviated in every case.

- *Disorders of the Immune System.* Cordyceps appears to be one of the most adaptive immunomodulators. The mushroom was found to quiet immune cells in patients with abnormally overactive immune systems, and to raise immune system functions in patients with low or compromised immunological activity. For example, researchers reported that patients with lupus, an auto-immune disease, had improved immune cell counts. Other scientists are experimenting with cordyceps in the treatment of HIV-positive patients.

- *Fatigue.* There are many indications for the use of cordyceps in the treatment of fatigue and weakness, and it is used by athletes and nonathletes of all age groups.

- *Cancer.* Significant improvements have been seen in patients with lung cancer who were treated with a combination of cordyceps and chemotherapy. In one study, researchers reported that cordyceps helped alleviate symptoms in 72 percent of patients. Problems such as fatigue, pain, fever, and vomiting were reduced by 50 percent and more, and there were significant increases in the T-cell activity of every patient.

  Researchers have found that cordyceps improves patients' tolerance to chemotherapy and radiation, and that it decreases the toxic effect on bone marrow caused by these conventional therapies. Patients taking cordyceps have a better chance of surviving cancer because cordyceps increases their ability to withstand conventional cancer therapies. In addition, ongoing laboratory research has suggested that cordyceps also acts as an antitumor agent and has been effective in fighting melanoma, leukemia, sarcoma, lymphoma, and other cancerous growths.

This book will provide you with in-depth information about the use of cordyceps for these and other medical disorders. Chapter 1 explores the history of the mushroom from its medicinal uses in ancient China to its discovery in recent years by Western scientists and herbalists. In Chapter 2, you will learn about the use of cordyceps in the treatment of heart disease. Specific ailments such as arrhythmia, chronic heart failure, and pulmonary heart disease are discussed in terms of their conventional treatments and their response to treatment with cordyceps. Although atherosclerosis is a heart-related disease, it is considered separately in Chapter 3. You will learn what cholesterol is, how it may cause atherosclerosis, and how cordyceps can help. Two major diseases of the liver, cirrhosis and hepatitis B, and the effectiveness of cordyceps in the treatment of these diseases are reviewed in Chapter 4. The succeeding chapter provides information about the successful use of cordyceps in treating the problem of sexual impotence in men, known as *erectile dysfunction*. Alternative therapies for this problem are also discussed. As we know from doctors of traditional Chinese medicine, cordyceps directly affects the kidneys and lungs, and they have long used cordyceps to treat disorders of these organs. Chapter 6 reviews three major kidney diseases and how they have responded to treatment with cordyceps. And in Chapter 7, you will learn how cordyceps can help patients suffering from lung and respiratory diseases. Since the onset of the AIDS epidemic, a great deal of research has been done on the immune system. Chapter 8 discusses the immune system and the successful use of cordyceps in treating disorders such as diabetes, cancer, and AIDS. Fatigue is a common problem that is often mis-diagnosed by doctors. In Chapter 9, we explore the effectiveness of cordyceps in alleviating two debilitating ailments—chronic fatigue and chronic fatigue syndrome. Finally, Chapter 10 will tell you how to buy cordyceps, what to look for, and how much you should take. There is also a resource section at the back of the book that lists some companies that sell cordyceps.

Whether you suffer from any of the problems discussed in this book or you are simply interested in learning more about this remarkable dietary supplement, *Cordyceps: China's Healing Mushroom* will provide you with information that may put you on the road to good health and well-being.

CHAPTER 1

THE STORY OF CORDYCEPS

*C*ordyceps sinensis belongs to a group of fungi that includes such delicacies as truffles and morels. It is a rare capless mushroom found at altitudes of 9,000 to 16,000 feet in the moist alpine meadows of the Himalayas and other high mountain ranges in Tibet and China. The mushroom feeds off a rare type of cold-temperature caterpillar that hibernates just below the surface of the frozen ground until it becomes a solid mummified form, completely composed of the mushroom.

We know that doctors in China and other Asian countries have used cordyceps as a healing agent for at least 1,000 years. But in recent years, the mushroom has found its way into alternative and conventional Western medicine. One reason for this is the modernization of production techniques, which has increased production and availability and has lowered the price of this ancient and versatile herbal remedy.

HOW CORDYCEPS IS GROWN

Recent scientific advances have literally brought the mush-

room down from the mountains. Using cell-culture technology, researchers have found a way to grow cordyceps
commercially without the rare caterpillars. In fact, many
of the medical findings concerning the use of cordyceps
were made possible following the discovery of techniques
for producing the section of the mushroom called the
mycelium. The mycelium, which looks like white muslin, is
the part of the mushroom found beneath the soil, in old
leaves, and in decaying wood. When it's dried, it bears a
striking resemblance to tofu, only with a stringy, thread-
like texture. As the mycelium matures, it forms a complete
mushroom.

It has been discovered that the medicinal properties of
cultured mycelia are equally effective as those of cordyceps
mushrooms found in the wild. In fact, given the right
nutrients, environment, and other conditions, the cordyceps mycelium has virtually the same biological activity as
the wild form of the mushroom.

Mycelia can be grown in much the same way as the
yeasts used in baking and brewing are grown. Modern
processes for growing mycelia are extremely technical.
Huge electronically controlled culture systems guarantee
optimum levels of the natural constituents and keep out
any foreign substances that could potentially contaminate
the growth process. When the growth cycle reaches the
desired point, the mycelia are dried in a germ-free environment to produce a sterile brown powder for encapsula-
tion. In sharp contrast to the price of the rare, wild mushroom—currently as high as $1,000 per pound—the success-
ful production of mycelia has greatly reduced the cost of
cordyceps and, consequently, has increased their availability. The benefits to consumers are considerable. Today,
cordyceps can be found in pharmacies and health-food
stores in many countries, whereas not too long ago, it
would have been far too expensive for most consumers to
even consider buying.

A BRIEF HISTORY OF CORDYCEPS

The first document concerning *Cordyceps sinensis* was written in AD 620 during the Tang Dynasty. For thousands of years the only descriptions of cordyceps were those of the ancient Chinese who alluded to the existence of a strange organism with the amazing ability to transform itself into a plant and then back again into an animal. For all anyone knew, the plant was purely mythical. But following the more recent scientific interest in cordyceps by China's scientific community, we now know a great deal about the use of the mushroom and what the ancient herbal texts had to say. For instance, it turns out that cordyceps was used to treat hiccups, and sometimes it was soaked in yellow wine to make a tonic for the kidneys and for the relief of pain in the groin and knees. Cordyceps was also prepared with duck following a recipe that seems to have been intended mainly for the elderly. According to one of the older Chinese texts, the dish was prepared for convalescing patients. It was believed that the mushroom produced a tonic effect equivalent to taking 30 grams of ginseng. Another text explains that cordyceps cooked with duck was fed to people who were recuperating after a severe illness or suffering from cancer or fatigue.

But cordyceps was prepared with all kinds of meats. One recipe called for lean pork cooked with cordyceps for the relief of fatigue, sexual impotence, or weak kidneys. Cooked with steamed turtle, cordyceps was said to be good for treating sexual and reproductive problems in men and women. The same recipe was prescribed to alleviate the symptoms of fatigue, tuberculosis, and hemorrhoids.

Western Interest in Cordyceps

In 1723, a Jesuit priest from Paris named Father Perennin Jean Baptiste du Halde collected specimens of the plant in

China and brought them home to France. Three years later, cordyceps became the first mushroom associated with insects to be described in a European publication. The illustration accompanying the article by French physicist René de Réaumur was a simple rendering of a caterpillar with a twig-like growth sprouting from its head. It was a fantastic discovery for the time. In Europe, it led to the use of microorganisms to control crop pests. And naturalists soon arrived at the idea of using the mushroom as a natural biological control.

For eighteenth-century Europeans, nature was full of surprises, and for those concerned with medicine, the mystery plant became quite alluring. They learned that the cordyceps was highly valued as an herbal medicine in China—in fact, the Emperor's own physicians were prescribing it. The same Jesuit priest who had carried the mushroom to France brought the news of cordyceps as a medicinal food to Europe. Father Perennin wrote that the "roots" of these rare plants were highly esteemed by Chinese nobles, "not only because of their miraculous changes, but from possessing the virtues of ginseng."[1] The Emperor's physicians told the priest that they only used the plant at the palace in Peking because it was so difficult to obtain. Costing four times its weight in silver, the mushroom had to be imported from far away in the mountainous kingdom of Tibet and adjoining regions, and it was available only in small quantities.

During his stay in China, Father Perennin had kept a record of events concerning cordyceps. Apparently, its true nature wasn't revealed to him all at once. In his diary, he laments that he hasn't been successful in getting a full account of the shape of the leaves, the color of the flower, or the height of its stalk. But from his writings, it's obvious that the medicinal properties of the plant were what really interested him. He learned that the mysterious plant was able to fortify the body and restore it to health. In one passage of his journal, he notes that cordyceps can "strengthen and renovate the powers of the system that have been reduced either by overexertion or long sickness."[2]

Upon returning to France, Father Perennin published an account of the effects of the plant on his own health. He wrote that during one cold rainy season in China, he had become extremely debilitated. He had lost his appetite and couldn't sleep, and in spite of having taken all sorts of remedies from the locals, his health was no better. But a chance visit from an acquaintance changed everything. The visitor was an official envoy to the Emperor on his way to pay tribute at the Great Palace in Peking, and he had brought along some cordyceps. Extremely concerned about the priest's poor health, he strongly recommended that he take it. According to Perennin, he had to take 8.5 grams of the whole cordyceps mushroom with the caterpillar casing still attached, stuff it into the belly of a freshly killed duck, and then boil the duck over a slow fire. Once the duck had been boiled, he had to remove the cordyceps and eat the duck meat every morning and evening for eight or ten days. He wrote that after trying the experiment, his appetite returned and his health was restored.

The Dissemination of Cordyceps

Details about the use of cordyceps for medicinal purposes were published during the Ching Dynasty in mid-eighteenth-century China. Nearly one hundred years later, cordyceps was imported by Japanese herbalists, who called the mushroom *totsu kasu* or *tochukaso*, meaning "summer grass, winter worm." The Japanese name derives from the old Chinese word for the mushroom, *hia tsao tong tchong*, which means "winter worm, summer plant." The common name currently used in China is *dongchongxiacao*, or *chongcao* for short.

By 1918, cordyceps was for sale in most American cities

with any sizeable Chinese population. In fact, there are records from as far back as the middle 1800s indicating that Chinese doctors were practicing their traditional medicine in Idaho and Oregon, and they were using cordyceps successfully for the treatment of arthritis, respiratory and digestive diseases, infections of the reproductive organs, and cardiovascular diseases.

Identification of the mythical plant-animal wasn't officially cleared up until 1843, when the *New York Journal of Medicine* reported that the mystery of the "insect-plant" had been solved. Reverend Dr. M.J. Berkeley had discovered that the "root" of the cordyceps plant was indeed a caterpillar, but its entire body was a hardened mass consisting almost entirely of the cordyceps mushroom. Nothing remained of the caterpillar except a micro-thin remnant of its outermost form. Inside was a hard, dense mass of white mushroom mycelium.

Around the turn of the nineteenth century, the top producer of herbal medicines in the United States was a company run by the Lloyd brothers of Cincinnati, Ohio. Curtis Gates Lloyd, a mushroom botanist, had arranged for the publication of a letter about cordyceps from a professor in China named N. Gist Gee. His letter explained that cordyceps was carried down from the mountains of Tibet by tribespeople who made their collections at 12,000 to 15,000 feet. Gee wrote that the mushroom part of the plant was black, whereas the caterpillar part appeared yellowish. During the winter, the caterpillar was said to live in the soil and move about like a silkworm. Its body was covered with hair. During the summer, the hair grew out of the surface of the soil, and the entire creature turned to grass. "If it is not taken, the grass will again turn into a [creature] in the winter."

Professor Gee explained that in China cordyceps was a valuable medicine used for the treatment of jaundice, asthma, and serious injuries. Chinese doctors also recognized that is was "good for protecting the lungs, enriching the kidneys, stopping the flowing or spitting of blood, decomposing phlegm produced from persistent coughing, and curing consumption." He went on to relate that cordyceps had been used as a tonic in Chinese medicine for the previous 1,000 years and was taken with duck meat or beaten into a powder and mixed with other natural tonics. In one example, he wrote, "When boiled with pork, [cordyceps] is employed as an antidote for opium poisoning and as a cure for opium eating." He added that "with pork and chicken, it is taken as a tonic and mild stimulant by convalescent persons and rapidly restores them to health and strength."[3]

Cordyceps Research

Research on cordyceps has been extensive in China. The result is that today there are a number of mycelial products on the market. Each has a different name and special conditions for successful growth. The most developed and extensively studied strain of the cordyceps mycelium is grown in a basic medium composed of soybean. It is called Cs-4 *(Paecilomyces hepiali)*. Other strains of cordyceps mycelia include *Paecilomyces sinensis* and *Cephalosporium sinensis*. The Latin names designate the strains, which are not identical even though they share the same parent mushroom, *Cordyceps sinensis*.

In 1972, researchers at the Institute of Materia Medica of the Chinese Academy of Medical Sciences began a ten-year project collecting and analyzing wild cordyceps from nearly every part of China. Because cordyceps is rare and very difficult to collect, the researchers' goal was to develop a superior strain of the mushroom to supply increasing worldwide demand for cordyceps. The strain of cordyceps they developed, tested, and finally decided on is known as *Cordyceps Cs-4*, or simply Cs-4.

Cordyceps Cs-4 was selected from among 200 other strains of the mushroom. It was isolated from the natural cordyceps found in the Province of Qinghai, an area that for millennia has been renowned for the mushroom. It was chosen because it is closest to the wild mushroom in the similarity of its chemical components and in its beneficial qualities as an herbal medicine. In fact, there are almost no differences between the two varieties of mushrooms. Furthermore, Cs-4 meets rigorous standards of safety, can grow rapidly in a variety of media, and resists contamination. In 1987, China's Ministry of Public Health approved Cs-4—or *jinshuibao,* as it is called in China—for use by the general population. Later, it became the first traditional Chinese medicine to be approved under the country's new and stringent medical standards. In the United States, this strain is available under the product name *CordyMax Cs-4* by Pharmanex.

Unless I am obliged to refer to a particular strain of cordyceps, I have chosen to use the general terms *cordyceps* and *mycelium* throughout this book.

CONCLUSION

Cordyceps has come a long way since the days of ancient Chinese discovery and modern scientific rediscovery. Widespread availability of the affordable, commercially cultured mycelium marks a new beginning for cordyceps. You can now find cordyceps in the supplement section of many health-food stores and pharmacies in the United States and through direct mail. Some people may try the product for very specific reasons, and others for general health. Whatever the reason, as you read the information in this book, you will learn that the powers of cordyceps are not easily categorized. Indeed, you will discover that the plant can be helpful in a great variety of ways.

CHAPTER 2

CORDYCEPS AND HEART DISEASE

In traditional Chinese medicine, cordyceps is known as an herbal medicine that goes to the meridians of the lungs and kidneys. It is believed that cordyceps invigorates the kidneys and protects the lungs. Based on its use as a lung-specific medicine, doctors of traditional Chinese medicine, or TCM, reasoned that it could also benefit the heart. In study after study, they found that cordyceps produced excellent results in the treatment of arrhythmia, chronic heart failure, and pulmonary heart disease. Before we discuss the value of cordyceps in treating these disorders, let's describe the heart and its function in terms of Western and traditional Chinese medicine.

THE FUNCTION OF THE HEART

The heart is an extraordinary pump. The amount of electromagnetic energy it produces is 1,000 times that of the brain. In fact, its energy is so strong that it can be picked up by a magnetometer placed at a distance of several feet from the body. Doctors now recognize that the heart secretes hormones that have a balancing effect on the cardiovascular system.

It seems that the heart has only begun to yield its secrets. Scientific evidence indicates that the heart sends sensory data to the brain. Our emotional state has a direct impact on the electrical rhythms generated by the heart, and these rhythms are sent back to the brain through the autonomic nervous system. Other findings suggest that the heart has its own nervous system that operates semi-independently of the central nervous system. Referred to as the *cardiac nervous system,* it produces electrical rhythms that affect the immune system and the brain. These rhythms can help doctors monitor a patient's risk of sudden death from heart failure.

VIEWS OF HEART DISEASE

Doctors of traditional Western and Eastern medicine have always viewed disease from different perspectives. This is reflected in the way they research and treat numerous illnesses, even extremely serious disorders such as heart disease. In recent years, however, Western doctors have broadened their horizons.

Traditional Western Medicine's View of Heart Disease

Research into the leading cause of death in the Western world has undergone a revolution of sorts. Western doctors have a far more extensive understanding of the causes and effects of heart disease than ever before. As a result, the treatment of heart disease is now much more holistic than it was in the past.

Some researchers are beginning to investigate the effects of worry on the heart. A recent study concludes that the type of worries a patient has can affect the outcome of heart disease. For example, one long-term study in older men found a strong association between coronary artery heart disease and persistent worries about social conditions such as economic recession. The researchers concluded that older men who are chronic worriers may be at greater risk for this disease. This suggests that broader psychosocial factors must be examined in assessing individual risks for heart disease. If a relationship between chronic worrying and coronary heart disease is established, then patients may be advised to receive some form of psychotherapy, such as meditation or talk therapy, dietary changes, and physical exercise.

In 1996, researchers in Finland made a breakthrough in the study of the effects of stress on the body. They questioned sixty-nine healthy middle-aged men to determine their levels of "vital exhaustion," which was defined by their positive answers to questions regarding lack of energy and feelings of fatigue, sadness, demoralization, and irritability. Factors of lifestyle were not considered in the study. Doctors found that long-term stress can increase levels of substances produced in our blood plasma that may increase our risk of developing clogged arteries. Their finding gives added support to the belief that stress kills.

Researchers are now looking more closely at incidences of heart attack and the possible contribution of bacteria called *Chlamydia pneumoniae*, which are passed through coughing and sneezing. The bacteria get into the lungs and cause a flu-like disease of the upper respiratory tract, which can progress to pneumonia. Additional evidence suggests that these bacteria also cause atherosclerosis, or damage to the walls of the arteries. This in turn causes the formation of clots that impair normal blood circulation, which can cause heart attacks. By studying animals infected with *Chlamydia pneumoniae*, researchers found that the bacteria can invade artery tissues, even tissues of the main artery of the heart. In one experiment, more than half the test animals developed the telltale lesions known as arterial plaques, which can grow and lead to heart attacks. (See Chapter 3 for an in-depth discussion of atherosclerosis.)

Traditional Chinese Medicine's View of Heart Disease

Before discussing traditional Chinese medicine, I must point out that I was trained in Western medicine and still find the Chinese traditional system fairly abstract. For me, it represents a completely different medical language. Relatively few physicians trained in Western medicine have enough time or interest in TCM to learn the basics. But since educating myself about cordyceps, I have become much more open-minded. I also realize that many readers will want to know about the traditional Chinese side of the equation.

It has been said that traditional Chinese medicine attempts to understand the body as an ecosystem, a microcosm or small component of nature. The medical terminology that is used in TCM is based on the workings of nature. Water, air, wood, metal, fire, heat, cold, moisture, dryness, and dampness are some of the more common terms. These are metaphors for dynamic processes, and they are used to describe disease conditions in the body and to select appropriate treatments according to the individual needs of the patient.

Doctors of traditional Chinese medicine describe disease processes in terms of the state of the affected organs. For example, they diagnose heart disease according to the heart's state of congestion or depletion, and either state indicates a conflict with the lungs and kidneys. Furthermore, ancient Chinese medical texts represented the main organs of the body with pictograms that reflected the belief that they are entire systems in and of themselves, each having its own energy. This is also why words such as Lung and Kidney are often capitalized in translations of Chinese texts.

COMMON DISEASES OF THE HEART

The heart is the center of the cardiovascular system, which also includes arteries, veins, and capillaries. It is an extremely complex system that is directly linked to the lungs and the pulmonary system. There are numerous disorders of the heart. Some involve a failure of the heart itself. Others involve a failure of one or more of the systems that work in conjunction with the heart. In the following sections, I will discuss three common heart disorders and how they have responded in clinical tests involving cordyceps.

Cardiac Arrhythmia

Cardiac arrhythmia is simply a disturbed or abnormal heartbeat or rhythm. The most common type of arrhythmia, *atrial fibrillation,* currently affects over two million people the United States. In older individuals, hypertension (high blood pressure), cardiac surgery, and coronary artery disease cause 65 percent of all arrhythmias. Individuals afflicted with arrhythmia are at an exceptionally high risk for stroke, estimated to be five times the normal rate. Atrial fibrillation is thought to cause approximately 15 to 20 percent of the 500,000 strokes that occur in the United States each year.

Arrhythmia has many causes. Medical researchers list factors such as lack of oxygen, acute intoxication, hyperthyroidism, rheumatic valvular disease, artificial heart valves, bypass tracts, severe congestive heart failure, heart attacks, and other heart-related disorders. Arrhythmias, even potentially fatal ones, can also be caused by metabolic disorders such as hypothermia and acidosis, a condition that can result from kidney disease. Some medications can increase the risk of arrhythmias. Among them are cardiovascular agents, antipsychotic drugs, certain antidepressants and drug combinations, and extremely high doses of stimulants such as nicotine or caffeine.

There is a great need for more effective treatments and means of preventing arrhythmias. Unfortunately, many drug therapies for arrhythmia are associated with major risks. These include heart failure and even the worsening of certain kinds of arrhythmias, which can require the use of pacemakers. Recent studies indicate that blood anticoagulants such as aspirin and warfarin may help prevent stroke in arrhythmia patients aged sixty to seventy-five.

Cordyceps and Arrhythmia

In 1990, a clinical study of wild cordyceps in the treatment of thirty-seven arrhythmia patients was conducted by the Department of Internal Medicine at Hunan Medical University. The researchers reported that nineteen patients were cured—six within the first week and another thirteen within two to three weeks—and eleven of the remaining patients showed some improvement.

A larger study of 200 patients was undertaken in China at Guangzhou Medical College. Patients with arrhythmia took 1,500 milligrams of cordyceps per day for a period of two weeks. An incredible 74.5 percent of patients showed improvement with cordyceps. And in 1994, another clinical trial involving thirty-eight elderly patients also reported excellent results. In this study, patients took 3,000 milligrams of cordyceps every day for three months. In a group of twenty-four patients diagnosed with a type of arrhythmia called *supraventricular* arrhythmia, twenty patients showed clinical improvement, and their electrocardiograms, or ECGs, showed partial or complete recovery. Patients with *ventricular* arrhythmia partially improved or completely recovered ECG patterns in eight of ten cases. The medical status of three patients who had complete blockage of the right branch of the cardiac nervous system also changed for the better. Researchers concluded that the positive effects of cordyceps increase over time—the longer patients take it, the more their medical condition improves.

A clinical trial in 1994 to determine the effectiveness of cordyceps in treating ventricular arrhythmia produced promising results. This time, researchers used more stringent measures by comparing a group given a placebo with a group given the cordyceps. Neither the researchers nor the patients knew who was taking cordyceps and who was taking the placebo. This more infallible kind of study, known as a *double-blind placebo-controlled trial*, is the preferred scientific method in Western medicine for the study of new drugs and herbal medicines. After randomly assigning each of the sixty-four patients to one of the two groups, researchers gave each patient in the test group 1,500 milligrams of cordyceps every day for two weeks. When the trial was unblinded, the results in the cordyceps group were remarkable. More than 80 percent of patients in the cordyceps group partially or completely recovered, whereas only 10 percent of patients in the placebo group showed similar improvement. The remaining patients showed no change in their conditions.

Chronic Heart Failure

Although we are still not certain about the causes of chronic heart failure, we do know the signs. The pumping action of the heart becomes dysfunctional, usually because the heart has been damaged in some way. Consequently, the body retains water and salt, which results in a reduction in cardiac performance. Eventually, fluid leaks into the lungs and/or the lower part of the body, which causes edema, fatigue, and difficulty breathing. In an effort to compensate for these changes, the body retains fluids to help maintain pressure in the tissues. Finally, the arteries become constricted, and this puts more of a burden on the heart, which then becomes arrhythmic.

When the heart is in a chronic state of failure, it can't support the skeletal muscles. And for this reason, patients with chronic heart failure often develop abnormal skeletal muscle tissue, which decreases their bulk, strength, and endurance. In addition, exchanges of oxygen and carbon dioxide in the lungs can't always be maintained, and some patients show increased bronchial sensitivity.

Chronic heart failure patients who have already had at least one heart attack have a two- to four-times greater risk of dying from another heart attack. About one-third of patients die from circulatory failure, and approximately another one-third die suddenly. Short of a heart transplant, chronic heart failure is treated with various combinations of diuretics, digoxin, calcium antagonists, beta blockers, and *ACE inhibitors*, which dilate the blood vessels. Diuretics are the primary treatment, and no one in Western medicine has come up with a better alternative. In chronic heart failure, diuretics seem to enhance the full capacity of the veins to carry blood unimpeded, and they help the body control the retention of water and salt.

One approach to preventing the recurrence of heart attacks in patients with chronic heart failure is the use of blood-thinning agents. Nevertheless, a group of researchers at the University of Glasgow concluded that no single drug is likely to be effective, at least for the majority of patients, because chronic heart failure is a multifaceted syndrome. Hopefully, future treatments will be found to address the underlying disease rather than the myriad of symptoms it presents.

A review of the major clinical trials in chronic heart disease concluded that although some advances have been made in increasing the lifespan of patients, the outlook remains bleak. The same conclusion was reached by the European Society of Cardiology. Doctors are now placing greater emphasis on preventing and slowing the progression of the disease. They also recognize that no single approach can manage all chronic heart failure problems, and treatments must be designed in accordance with the needs of each individual case.

There is increasing interest in exercise training as part of the treatment for this disease. Research suggests that appropriate training can improve the capacity for exercise in chronic heart failure patients, decrease their overly active sympathetic nervous system, and improve skeletal muscle tissue. We know that exercise therapy increases the body's ability to use oxygen and decreases the abnormal burning of sugar stores. It is now widely accepted that inactivity leads to greater deterioration in people with chronic heart failure. This is a remarkable development. After all, it wasn't so long ago that doctors were warning chronic heart failure patients to avoid exercise. Of course, not every patient can safely participate in exercise training; but for those with less severe cases of chronic heart failure, exercise and a more active lifestyle are now commonly suggested for strengthening skeletal muscles and improving quality of life.

Cordyceps and Chronic Heart Failure

Cordyceps for the treatment of chronic heart failure has been the subject of many studies, and the results are very promising. One of the longest clinical studies ever conducted with cordyceps lasted for twenty-six months and was completed in 1995. Researchers at Fu-Jian Medical College in China set out to test cordyceps for its potential effects on the quality of life of sixty-four patients with chronic heart failure. Patients were randomly assigned to a control group of thirty patients who received conventional Western medicines alone and a test group of thirty-four patients who received a daily dosage of 3 to 4 grams of cordyceps in addition to the conventional Western medicines. Patients were regularly checked for changes in their ECGs, quality of life, and other factors according Western medical standards.

Although there was no important difference between the number of patients who died in each of the two groups, investigators noted differences in all other areas. In the categories of shortness of breath and fatigue, patients taking cordyceps improved by an average of 66 percent, whereas the control group improved by an average of 25 percent. Statistically significant progress showed up in the cordyceps group in cardiac output, stroke volume, and heartbeat.

Measurable recovery was found in levels of general physical activity in twelve of the thirty control-group patients, whereas twenty-seven of thirty-four patients in the cordyceps group made similar progress. In addition, patients taking cordyceps reported a greater sense of general well-being, an increase in self-control, a decrease in symptoms of depression and anxiety, and an increase in sexual desire. The researchers concluded that cordyceps is beneficial to patients with chronic heart failure, especially in terms of their quality of life.

Pulmonary Heart Disease

As its name suggests, pulmonary heart disease involves problems in the respiratory tract. In these cases, an otherwise healthy heart becomes impaired because of a persistent disorder of the lungs, bronchi, or other respiratory organs. Prolonged defective pulmonary function may increase the workload on the heart and eventually cause heart failure.

The disease is found most often in elderly patients who have repeatedly suffered from emphysema, chronic bronchitis, or bronchial asthma. Long-term poor nutrition may also be a factor. Pulmonary heart disease often reaches an acute stage when patients develop a bacterial infection in the respiratory tract as the result of catching a cold. If the airways have been obstructed with phlegm for a long time, the condition leads to chronic deficiency of oxygen. Infection of the respiratory tract is more likely to occur in older patients whose illness has run a long course and whose immune systems have been weakened.

At the cellular level, the energy factories in the heart cells known as the *mitochondria* undergo a change in their metabolic function. When resting, older mitochondria frequently make sufficient amounts of a substance called ATP, or *adenosine triphosphate,* which provides the heart with all the fuel it needs. But old mitochondria are not always able to get this fuel directly into the tank. Exactly what happens at this stage is not yet completely understood. However, we do know that the problem further impedes the heart's ability to respond to stress and to keep its metabolic functions within a normal range.

In conventional treatment, diuretics are given to reduce the workload on the heart. Additional therapies such as oxygen and antibiotics are prescribed to correct electrolyte and acid-base imbalances and to correct low nutrient levels due to diminished appetite.

Cordyceps and Pulmonary Heart Disease

The Department of Medicine at Shandong Provincial Hospital in China recently conducted a study of cordyceps in the treatment of acute pulmonary heart disease in fifty patients. These were challenging cases. Ranging in age from thirty-eight to eighty, the patients had been diagnosed with pulmonary heart disease and other complications.

In traditional Chinese medicine, patients with long-term pulmonary heart disease are usually diagnosed with a "deficiency syndrome" of the lungs and kidneys and with "exhaustion of vital essence." In selecting cordyceps, TCM doctors were adhering to the principle of curing the kidneys before treating asthma, which has some similarities to pulmonary heart disease.

Poor nutrition seems to be common in patients with pulmonary heart disease. One study estimates that more than 90 percent of pulmonary heart disease patients are malnourished in one way or another. Researchers contend that malnutrition lowers patients' immunity and exacerbates their heart condition because it weakens the respiratory muscles. Consequently, asthmatic symptoms, coughing, sleep disturbance, and an already poor mental state become more severe. Let's look at the particulars of this study.

The thirty patients in the control group received oxygen by way of a nasal tube and intravenous antibiotics for thirty days. The test group of twenty patients received the same treatments plus 1,000 milligrams of cordyceps three times a day for thirty days. By the end of the study, it was clear that the cordyceps group fared much better than the control group. There were positive changes in patients' heart and respiratory functions, productive cough, shortness of breath, mental state, and sleep. In all, improvement was evident in 94 percent of patients in the cordyceps group. In comparison, the improvement rate in the control group was a little over 60 percent. Given that the cases chosen for this study were at an acute stage, these results are notable. The doctors who conducted the study commented that along with the ease of administering the cordyceps, their results in achieving a relatively favorable outcome with the routine Western treatment warranted a much wider complementary use of cordyceps in treating pulmonary heart disease.

This study demonstrates the versatility of cordyceps. In fact, a significantly greater number of patients who took cordyceps plus Western medications reported that they experienced less depression and anxiety than those who only took Western drugs. This may indicate another kind of activity, perhaps even an antidepressive one. In addition, patients' sexual-function index was one-and-one-half times that of the routine treatment group, which was reflected in the 92-percent effective rate of improvement in mental state versus the 60-percent rate in the routine group. The 96-percent improvement rate in sleep experienced by the cordyceps group may be another reflection of antidepressant activity.

CONCLUSION

Patients suffering from various types of heart disease react extremely well when they are put on programs involving a blending of Eastern and Western medicine. It is clear that Western medicine can be highly effective in controlling the damaging effects of heart disease. But Western medicine combined with cordyceps has been proven be even more effective. As we saw in the results of the Shandong study, when cordyceps is combined with traditional Western medicine, the results are often remarkable. It is therefore tempting to suggest that cordyceps may play a significant role in helping prevent and treat heart diseases.

CHAPTER 3

CORDYCEPS AND ATHEROSCLEROSIS

Although atherosclerosis is considered a heart-related disorder involving the cardiovascular system, it is given special treatment in this chapter because the disease is so widespread in the United States and other Western countries. As we will see, its development is closely linked to cholesterol levels, and it is highly preventable.

Every week, we hear or read something in the news about the need to lower our cholesterol levels in order to achieve optimal health. As you know, diet plays a significant role in cholesterol management; and for this reason, it can be difficult for some people to lower their cholesterol levels. Instead of developing such a high level of cholesterol that prescription drugs are warranted, people can take supplements that make a notable difference when combined with exercise and a well-balanced diet. Cordyceps is one of these supplements.

High cholesterol levels in the body can lead to many medical disorders, and atherosclerosis is one of the most common and serious of these problems. Before we discuss the use of cordyceps in turning back the clock on atherosclerosis, it will help to understand what cholesterol is and what we mean by high cholesterol levels.

WHAT IS CHOLESTEROL?

Although there are different types of cholesterols, the general term cholesterol refers to a fatty, wax-like substance produced mainly by the liver and used by the body to help it perform vital functions such as cell renewal and hormone production. The liver makes most of the cholesterol the body needs for survival, but cholesterol is also present in animal products. A diet high in saturated fats can contribute to high cholesterol levels.

Types of Cholesterol

The body needs certain forms of cholesterol in order to function properly. But an overabundance of some types of cholesterol can be harmful. For this reason, you often hear the terms "good cholesterol" and "bad cholesterol." *High-density lipoprotein cholesterol,* or HDL cholesterol, is a type that many of us could use more of. Generally speaking, there is a strong correlation between high levels of HDL cholesterol and low incidences of atherosclerosis. In addition, disorders such as diabetes, hypertension, and obesity are usually found in connection with low levels of HDL cholesterol. It's likely that HDL cholesterol protects the body by transporting fats, or lipids, through the body. But *low-density lipoprotein cholesterol,* or LDL cholesterol, tends to deposit fats in the body. When fat is deposited on blood vessel walls, it can cause atherosclerosis. And when it is deposited in the liver, it can cause fatty liver tissue. Rigorous exercise, certain food supplements, and a diet rich in fish produce higher levels of HDL. The following list summarizes the characteristics of the different types of cholesterol.

❑ LDL, or Low-Density Lipoprotein Cholesterol:

- Is taken up by the liver

- Increases its levels in blood plasma when the liver can't process it as a result of a high dietary intake of cholesterol

- Becomes "foam cells" that adhere to arteries when they are taken up by *macrophages*—white blood cells whose job is to destroy and digest foreign microbes in the body

- Is made up of 50 percent cholesterol, 20 percent phospholipid, and 25 percent protein

❑ VLDL, or Very Low-Density Lipoprotein Cholesterol:

- Is secreted by the liver; also secreted by the intestines during fasting

- Is synthesized by the liver and turns into IDL cholesterol, and finally LDL cholesterol

- Contains 50 percent triglycerides, 30 percent cholesterol, and 20 percent phospholipids, of which 9 percent is protein

❑ IDL, or Intermediate-Density Lipoprotein Cholesterol:

- Are processed by liver for incorporation by cells

- Becomes LDL cholesterol when further metabolized by the liver

❑ HDL, or High-Density Lipoprotein Cholesterol:

- Is secreted by the intestines or liver

- Can form from metabolized VLDLs

- May be removed from system by the kidneys

- Contributes to healthy cholesterol levels

How Cholesterol Is Measured

Cholesterol levels are measured in terms of the total amount of cholesterol found in the blood, the amount of HDL, and/or the amount of LDL found in the blood. High total cholesterol is any amount over 200 mg/dL—that is, 200 milligrams of cholesterol in every deciliter of blood. A total cholesterol reading over 240 mg/dL is considered a high risk factor for cardiovascular diseases. HDL cholesterol levels below 35 mg/dL also contribute to cardiovascular disorders. And levels of 60 mg/dL or higher can decrease incidences of *coronary heart disease,* which occurs when there are obstructions in the coronary arteries. What is the connection between high levels of cholesterol and the development of atherosclerosis? The best way to answer this question is to explain what atherosclerosis is and how it develops.

WHAT IS ATHEROSCLEROSIS?

Atherosclerosis involves the formation of fatty deposits on the artery walls, which leads to their scarring, and finally to their thickening and hardening. The disorder develops over time and is closely linked to lifestyle and diet. For this reason, atherosclerosis is not an inevitable result of aging. Knowing how it develops can help us learn how to change or even reverse its course.

Atherosclerosis can develop when excess fat is stored in the body. Over time, the amount of fat in the blood can reach unhealthy levels, and the lining of the arteries runs a risk of developing deposits of fibrous plaques. These are essentially lesions or abrasions in the artery wall formed from fatty deposits that attract various cells of the immune system. Once these cells begin to attach themselves to the plaque, they bore into the inner wall of the arteries where they alter the normal cellular makeup to the point that the smooth-muscle cells of the arteries start to push inward. This starts a cycle of abnormal cell migration and the further accumulation of fatty cells, especially LDL cholesterol.

It gets worse. Immune system cells, particularly the macrophages, attack the LDL cholesterol in the plaque with blasts of free-radical electrons that oxidize the fat deposits. Oxidation produces more free-radical electrons, which can further damage artery walls. Antioxidant supplements such as vitamin E and green tea can help limit the destruction because they inhibit oxidation and the formation of free radicals. Cordyceps inhibits these radicals, too—a point we'll return to later.

Eventually, the accumulation of deposits enlarges the plaques. They can grow so large that they block the flow of blood to vital areas of the body, including the heart, brain, lower legs, and upper arms. In addition to droplets of cholesterol, the plaques attract immature immune cells and muscle cells that would normally have served to keep the arteries healthy and supple. The debris of cast-off cells on their way out of the system also gets stuck in these plaques. Eventually, the plaques grow to resemble scabs, which harden, crack, and develop crevices that trap even more cells. As a result, blood platelets begin to adhere and form large clumps known as *thrombi*. In time, they grow so hard that they become brittle and can break away and enter the bloodstream. This leaves a hole in the artery wall, which can result in hemorrhaging and sudden death.

Research and Treatment

The good news is that researchers are beginning to find ways of stabilizing and reducing these plaques by aggressively lowering levels of LDL cholesterol. The theory is that by lowering cholesterol levels, we can restore the inner lining of the arteries, which allows it to relax from the stiffened state it was in when burdened with plaques. One study of fourteen patients with atherosclerosis and mildly elevated LDL cholesterol found promising signs of plaque reversal. The patients in the University of California study were put on a two-year program of relaxation sessions, a vegetarian diet with a 12-percent fat intake, exercise training, and psychological and stress-management counseling. By the end of the study, all severe plaques in patients' arteries had regressed. However, only one in eight of the mild plaques had regressed, and the other half had progressed. This suggests the need to incorporate more measures or to supplement existing ones. The patients' LDL cholesterol levels were lowered by an average of 9 percent, and total cholesterol fell by a modest 13-percent average. Only three patients in the study required cholesterol-lowering prescription drugs.

Long-term studies have conclusively demonstrated that when cholesterol levels are lowered, the incidences of atherosclerosis and other heart diseases are substantially reduced. There is no doubt that atherosclerosis can be regressed in coronary heart disease patients by aggressively lowering levels of LDL cholesterol. In one study, the cholesterol-lowering agents *niacin* and *colestipol* reduced atherosclerotic conditions by 17 percent. Several of these studies have determined that aggressive therapy can result in a reduction in signs of coronary heart disease by as much as 89 percent.

Aside from prescription drugs, exercise can have a substantial effect on cholesterol levels. A study of twenty-six men with high cholesterol found that exercise training reduces levels of total cholesterol. The men, all forty-seven years old, were not asked to make changes in their diet; all they had to do was ride a stationary exercise bike three times a week. The duration of each exercise session varied according to the physical abilities of the individuals involved. Twenty-four weeks after beginning the exercise program, the men's cholesterol levels had dropped 9 percent. Despite these findings, total cholesterol levels are currently at or over 240 mg/dL in 30 percent of men and in 50 percent of women in the United States. It will take more than exercise to make any substantial difference.

Cordyceps and Atherosclerosis

Doctors in China have long believed that cordyceps helps blood circulation. Recent clinical studies have given a logical explanation to this belief by proving cordyceps to be a powerful cholesterol-lowering agent. The largest study of cordyceps for the treatment of high cholesterol was a clinical trial of 273 patients at nine hospitals in China. The trial excluded patients whose high cholesterol had resulted from diabetes mellitus, liver and liver-related diseases, kidney disease, and hypothyroidism. Patients received one gram (1,000 milligrams) of cordyceps three times a day. When they were tested after four or eight weeks, it was found that their cholesterol levels had dropped by an average of over 17 percent.

Cordyceps is used in China for the treatment of a type of *hyperlipidemia*—high levels of fat in the blood—that resists treatment with other agents. How it works is still not known, but it produces effects that are beneficial to people with high cholesterol. In two placebo-controlled trials, cordyceps reduced age-related oxidation of fats in patients aged sixty to eighty-four. After taking cordyceps, the patients' red blood cells had significantly higher levels of one of the body's natural antioxidants, an enzyme called *superoxide dismutase,* or SOD. In fact, SOD levels increased so much after the patients took cordyceps that they reached levels comparable to those of a group of young people aged seventeen to twenty, who were checked for comparison.

Increased levels of SOD activity are also found in elderly patients with chronic obstructive pulmonary disease and chronic kidney dysfunction taking cordyceps. These patients showed a significant decrease in cell-damaging free radicals known as *lipoperoxides*. Researchers can measure lipoperoxides in the form of a substance called *plasma malondialdehyde,* or MDA. In one study, patients taking cordyceps initially showed higher levels of MDA; but after three months of therapy, their levels equaled those found in seventeen- to twenty-year-olds. Why are these findings significant? Because they indicate that cordyceps reduces oxidative damage to cells. And these cells include those lining artery walls. Table 3.1 lists the results of treating high cholesterol with cordyceps.

Table 3.1. Cordyceps Mycelium in the Treatment of High Cholesterol

Year	1995	1995	1990
Duration of treatment	8 weeks	4 weeks	8 weeks
Number of patients	32	62	273
Total cholesterol	Decreased by 9.7 percent	Decreased by 16 percent	Decreased by 17.5 percent
HDL levels	Increased by 26.7 percent	Increased by 20 percent	Increased by 27.2 percent

Another way cordyceps helps prevent atherosclerosis is by decreasing the number of platelets that can get caught in the plaques. It does this by reducing the viscosity, or stickiness, of the blood. In a recent study, coronary heart disease patients who had taken 3 grams of cordyceps a day for three months showed a significantly decreased blood viscosity and a drop in total cholesterol of 21 percent.

CONCLUSION

Although cholesterol levels can be lowered by changes in diet and exercise, cordyceps has proven to be highly effective in lowering levels to an even greater extent. We now know that atherosclerosis can be prevented and, perhaps more important, it can be reversed. Whether cordyceps is combined with exercise and a well-balanced diet or with cholesterol-lowering prescription drugs, its health benefits are indeed dramatic and far-reaching.

CHAPTER 4

CORDYCEPS AND
THE LIVER

Research on cordyceps in the treatment of liver disease is still fairly new. Nonetheless, preliminary results of clinical tests with mycelium are almost certain to lead to its wider use, for there are compelling indications that cordyceps functions as a liver tonic. For example, when cordyceps is taken alone or in combination with other medicinal plants, it has proven to be beneficial to patients with *posthepatitis cirrhosis*. This is an often chronic liver disease resulting from inadequate healing of a liver infection caused by the hepatitis virus. As we will see, cordyceps is effective in treating hepatitis as well as cirrhosis. But first, let's review the functions of the liver according to the viewpoints of traditional Chinese and traditional Western medicine.

VIEWS OF THE LIVER

Traditional Chinese medicine uses an almost poetic language to describe the workings of the liver. This does not mean, however, that its description is inaccurate. In fact, the Eastern perspective serves to complement the Western perspective, which tends to be more matter-of-fact.

Traditional Chinese Medicine's View of the Liver

In traditional Chinese medicine, the liver is regarded as the organ system responsible for digestion and, odd as it may seem, for harmonizing the emotions. A relaxed, easygoing disposition is taken as a sign of liver harmony, whereas the opposite is generally regarded as a sign of liver disharmony, or even disease. According to TCM diagnostics, a sudden change in the emotions can affect the liver's health, which in turn can affect a person's emotional state. For example, anxiety and worry are thought to be damaging to the liver, which may be a good reason to take a more conscious role in controlling these feelings. It is also believed that the liver controls the ligaments, or tendons, and, to some degree, the muscles. Thus, an impaired ability to stretch and bend will also be seen as a problem related to the liver. A most curious view in TCM, especially to a Western-trained physician, links the eyes to the liver. Therefore, eye disorders are treated as liver problems.

In addition, doctors of traditional Chinese medicine believe that the liver is responsible for moving the blood and the *Qi* (pronounced *chee*), or life energy, throughout the body, and for regulating the body's activities. In fact, all activity depends on the Qi, whose movement is made smooth by the liver.

Traditional Western Medicine's Views of the Liver

Western medicine describes the liver in more mechanical terms and recognizes that its functions are numerous. The organ is located in the region of the upper right side of the abdomen. It stores and filters the blood, and it secretes the bile necessary for breaking down fats into very small, easily digestible units. The liver is the main site of fat synthesis and the source of cholesterol, of which about 30 percent is synthesized by the liver. The liver is also the source of blood glucose. It converts sugars into *glycogen,* which is stored in the liver and to a lesser extent in the muscles. Glycogen is turned into glucose and distributed to meet the body's energy requirements. Dietary sugars are either stored in the form of glycogen or turned into fatty acids, most of which are secreted by the liver in forms known as triglycerides, which are stored in our fatty tissues.

The liver is the only source of many of our plasma proteins and the main site where external and internal chemicals undergo transformation. Through transformative processes, it inactivates or detoxifies chemicals such as steroid hormones, toxins, and drugs and herbal medicines of all kinds before the body uses them. The liver also carries the burden of the toxic byproducts produced by these processes, and this can get the whole body into trouble.

CORDYCEPS AND LIVER DISEASES

It has been demonstrated that patients with certain liver diseases respond very well to cordyceps. Studies have been conducted on cordyceps and two major killers, cirrhosis and hepatitis of the liver. Let's take a look at these diseases separately.

Cirrhosis of the Liver

Cirrhosis is a degenerative disease of the liver in which healthy cells that are damaged by other problems such as hepatitis or excessive alcohol consumption are replaced by scar tissue. Although the disorder cannot be cured or reversed, its progress can be slowed or even stopped. Cirrhosis patients have 100 times the normal risk of developing liver cancer, and about 30 percent eventually die from liver complications such as liver cancer or chronic active hepatitis.

A recent study by Japanese and Chinese researchers found that mice developed a high-energy state of their livers, without signs of toxicity, after consuming large quantities of cordyceps mycelium. The researchers concluded that one of the main effects of taking cordyceps on a repeated basis might be a higher metabolic state of the liver. One drug prescribed to treat cirrhosis, called *malotilate*, helps the liver regenerate by activating the cells of its energy factories. This in turn boosts concentrations of an essential enzyme called ATP. The fact that cordyceps causes increases in ATP levels may be one way it helps repair the liver.

In 1986, an extract of cultured mycelium was tested in twenty-two patients with posthepatitis cirrhosis. Patients took 6,000 to 9,000 milligrams of cordyceps every day for three months, and by the end of the study, their symptoms had improved dramatically. Cirrhotic cells had disappeared in fifteen patients, and had decreased significantly in another six patients.

In one recent study, sixty-five patients with posthepatitis cirrhosis received cordyceps in addition to an extract of peach kernels, a traditional Chinese medicine used as a cough suppressant and also as a sedative for patients with high blood pressure. The results showed that cordyceps improved the function of various immunological cells. Abnormally raised levels of certain antibody proteins called *immunoglobulins* were lowered following the treatment, and levels of some antiviral antibodies were raised. Researchers concluded that cordyceps inhibits the hyperfunctional state of the immune system and increases positive immune-cell functions in posthepatitis cirrhosis patients. This is important because these changes correlate strongly with improvements in overall liver function.

Hepatitis B

The number of people currently infected with hepatitis B is thought to be more than 350 million worldwide. According to estimates from the World Health Organization, this number will soon reach 400 million. In most cases, hepatitis B is contracted from sexual contact and exposure to infected blood or needles. It is a leading cause of liver cancer, cirrhosis, and chronic hepatitis. Despite the availability of an effective vaccine, the disorder causes one million deaths a year. The problem is, the vaccine is too expensive in the very countries where the virus is most prevalent. The areas of highest occurrence are in Africa, Southeast Asia, and China. It has been estimated that over 8 percent of the population in these parts of the world are chronic carriers of the virus, and over 50 percent of the population will become infected during their lifetime. Although the figures are lower in the United States than they are in most countries, 1.25 million Americans are now suffering from chronic hepatitis B.

One of the biggest problems with hepatitis B is that even when the immune system is able to destroy infected cells and stop the virus from replicating, certain immune cells, known as *cytotoxic T lymphocytes,* may act against the virus without destroying infected cells in the liver. This means that something more must be done to prevent infected cells from becoming cancerous, especially in chronically infected people. The immunostimulating drug *alpha-interferon* is the main treatment for hepatitis B, but it's only effective in about 30 percent of cases, and it's very expensive.

Cordyceps can help treat many cases of hepatitis B. In one study, eighty-three patients who were carriers of the hepatitis-B virus, but who displayed no symptoms of the infection, were treated with cordyceps mycelium for three months. A complete conversion of antibodies to the virus was found in 33 of the test subjects, which indicates that the infection had been completely resolved and the virus was no longer contagious. In the same study, researchers reported that the number of antibodies positive for the virus had decreased in 47 percent of the patients. The patients ranged in age from two to fifteen, so their immune systems were not as developed as those of adults. This suggests that the benefits of cordyceps may be all the more significant. Why? Research has shown that the greater a person's immune response, the less likely he is to become a chronic hepatitis-B virus carrier. Only 3 to 5 percent of adults exposed to the virus become chronic carriers because their immune systems are fully developed. On the other hand, 95 percent of infected newborns become chronic carriers. And children under the age of six who are infected become chronic carriers of the virus in about 30 percent of cases.

A preliminary study in 1990 examined the benefits of cordyceps mycelium extract in thirty-two hepatitis-B patients. After three months of treatment with 3,750 milligrams of cordyceps a day, positive antibodies to the virus changed to negative in twenty-one patients, and tests showed liver function had improved or recovered completely in as many as twenty-three patients.

CONCLUSION

As we have seen, the combination of Eastern and Western medicines in the treatment of liver disease can have extremely positive results. And researchers have only begun to explore the potential of cordyceps in the fight against cirrhosis and hepatitis. There is no doubt that continued research will confirm what has already been learned—cordyceps can be instrumental in stopping the onslaught of these and other killer diseases.

CHAPTER 5

CORDYCEPS AND ERECTILE DYSFUNCTION

The widely accepted use of cordyceps in China as a sexual aid has barely raised an eyebrow from doctors in the West. But since investigating the old herbalists' tales myself, I can tell you that this is not something to be taken lightly. How cordyceps ever came to be used for sexual potency is not known with any certainty. Perhaps it was the shepherds in the high meadows of Tibet who witnessed the effect in their yaks from grazing among the grasses where the mushroom grows. Whatever the origin, historians believe that its use is hundreds if not thousands of years old. This belief is borne out by its mention in a number of ancient Chinese texts that refer to the use of cordyceps to cure impotence and implant sperm.

Sexual impotence in men is called *erectile dysfunction* or *male erectile disorder*. Erectile dysfunction is a recurring or persisting inability to achieve or maintain an erection sufficient enough to complete sexual activity. By one estimate, it affects one of every ten men of all ages. In the United States, a conservatively estimated 10 to 20 million men may have erectile dysfunction.

CAUSES OF ERECTILE DYSFUNCTION

One study on aging and sexual performance found that 5 percent of forty-year-old men suffered from total erectile dysfunction. In seventy-year-olds, the prevalence of total erectile dysfunction had tripled to 15 percent. And in a survey of American couples, 7 percent of the men, who were on average thirty-seven years old, complained that they had difficulty in getting an erection and 9 percent complained they had trouble keeping one. Although libido and the intensity of orgasms are generally thought to decrease as we grow older, age by itself is not a cause of erectile dysfunction. In men who are over fifty years old, more than 50 percent of cases of erectile disorder can be directly attributed to the buildup of atherosclerotic plaque in the blood vessels, including those in the penis. For at least half the men in this age group, high total cholesterol levels and low HDL cholesterol levels are associated with a greater incidence and increased risk of erectile dysfunction. In fact, one of the first indications of atherosclerosis in men is erectile dysfunction.

In diabetic men, there is a 28-percent probability that they will have some degree of erectile dysfunction. This is more than three times the 9-percent rate in the greater population. Men with type 1, or insulin-dependent, diabetes are predisposed to erectile dysfunction in part because their disease contributes to atherosclerosis. The small vessels of the arteries may develop a reduced capacity to supply blood to the main chamber in the penis. In addition, this disease may adversely affect the smooth muscles; and the autonomic nervous system, which is responsible for regulation and production of erections, may be damaged as well.

Older men who have blood-vessel disorders, or what we call *vascular disease,* and who are also chronic drinkers are even more prone to erectile dysfunction. Researchers suspect that the greater susceptibility among these men is due to a number of biochemical changes caused by alcohol. For example, a diseased liver takes up fewer male hormones and produces more female sex hormones, which can alter the balance of hormones that our bodies require for sexual function. This alteration may even be permanent. Alcohol consumption alone causes a reduction in testosterone production and in the concentration of testosterone in blood plasma. It also increases the rate at which testosterone is metabolized, and it alters the part of the brain responsible for the arousal process. Of course, there are many other causes of erectile dysfunction. They include stress, depression, and a number of physical disorders besides vascular diseases.

TREATMENT OPTIONS

There are many treatment options to correct erectile dysfunction, including talk therapy, chemical and hormonal therapy, and herbal remedies. In Western medicine, the use of prescriptions had been limited until the last twenty years. But today, Western medical therapy helps approximately 95 percent of men who experience erectile dysfunction. However, 5 to 6 percent of men find no relief from prescription treatments such as penile injections, vacuum devices, or prescription drugs. For many men, Western treatments may even have adverse side effects. Before we examine the treatment of erectile dysfunction with cordyceps, let's consider some conventional treatments for the disorder.

Surgery

Depending on the diagnostic criteria involved, reports indicate that a surgical technique known as *penile revascularization* is successful in 27 to 65 percent of cases involving

erectile dysfunction. Obviously, with this range of difference, not enough studies have been done to determine the
exact effectiveness of this surgery. The technique works
best for younger men who have suffered pelvic trauma.
However, in recent years, this and other surgical techniques are being re-evaluated, and drug therapy has all
but replaced them.

Drug Therapy

Drug therapy can involve prescription drugs as well as
nonprescription herbal remedies. All drugs that fall into
these two categories have some positive and some negative influence on the body. For example, treatment with
testosterone as a hormonal replacement therapy is one
method of helping some men, especially chronic alcohol
users with vascular disease. Nonetheless, there is a risk
that testosterone may increase symptoms of *prostatitis,* or
inflammation of the prostate. What's more, there is some
concern that increased testosterone levels may cause
prostate-cancer cells to multiply at a faster rate. A recent
study found that although testosterone enhances the sex
drive, it doesn't necessarily strengthen erectile capacity,
rigidity, or even sexual satisfaction.

Viagra, which is the name brand for *sildenafil citrate,* is a
temporary-acting drug that produces erections. It lasts for
only a few hours. Viagra works by allowing the smooth-
muscle cells inside the penis to relax, thereby allowing
increased blood flow. Although it's too soon to know precisely how many men can benefit from this latest "wonder
drug," some estimate that it is effective in 50 to 70 percent
of patients.

Viagra is not without dangerous side effects, however.
It can be fatal if an individual with a heart condition
takes it. In addition, some men have experienced impaired
vision, which can last up to twelve hours after taking the

drug. Therefore, it is essential that patients undergo a thorough medical examination before taking Viagra.

There are two well-known nonprescription drugs for erectile dysfunction that have been helpful to some men. The most widely recognized is a traditional African aphrodisiac called *yohimbine,* which comes from the bark of the yohimbe tree. But yohimbine can produce side effects and should only be taken under medical supervision. One study determined that yohimbine was effective in 34 percent of cases, and another study found that it was effective in helping 46 percent of men with erectile dysfunction.

The second nonprescription remedy is *muira puama,* a popular herbal aphrodisiac that comes from the Brazilian tree of the same name. Muira puama was said to be an effective sexual stimulant in 70 percent of volunteers who took the powdered, pinkish root. Although this herb and yohimbine can be used in the United States for the treatment of erectile dysfunction, they are not universally regarded as effective. In Germany, the government commission on herbal medicines states that their use is not recommended because of the risk of side effects and because there is not sufficient proof of their effectiveness. Yohimbine must not be taken by individuals with kidney or liver diseases or by those with chronic inflammatory conditions of the prostate or genitals.

Obviously, no single method of treatment can help everyone. In cases where erectile dysfunction has been brought on by psychological problems such as stress or depression, other therapies or medications may help. And cordyceps may well be the most promising and likely choice.

Cordyceps

Cordyceps, which acts on the libido over a period of weeks or months, can be classified as a sexual restorative. As I mentioned, its use as a remedy for sexual dysfunction has a long history in China. Cordyceps was simmered with other herbal medicines or cooked with meats such as lean pork, chicken, or steamed turtle, each of which was thought to have its own power to enhance sexual function.

Doctors of traditional Chinese medicine will tell you that cordyceps works by boosting the *jing*. From my Western point of view, the description of jing suggests something to do with the endocrine glands, which produce hormones. People believe that jing produces life and allows the organs to thrive. There are two forms of jing— the first type is inherited from one's parents as *congenital essence*; the second is developed after birth as *postnatal jing*—and the two forms reinforce each other. Postnatal jing, which is the basis of reproduction and development, is regarded as something dark, warm, and fluid-like. It is said that disharmonies of the jing are manifested in abnormal physical maturation, premature aging, sexual dysfunctions, reproductive difficulties, and congenital defects.

According to the precepts of TCM, if the jing and the Qi don't work at optimum efficiency, the brain can't function properly and mental health can't be achieved, which makes it impossible to have a healthy sex life. It is also believed that supplementing the kidneys with herbal mixtures that include cordyceps improves the body's resistance to disease, prevents premature aging, and strengthens sexual function. And because cordyceps helps the jing, the Qi, and the kidneys, it meets all the traditional Chinese medical requirements of a tonic suited to enhance sexual function.

Using Western scientific methods, researchers have determined that cordyceps stimulates activities in the body similar to those produced by the natural sex hormones. In 1995, laboratory research in Japan demonstrated that mycelium extract inhibits muscle contractions of the double chamber inside the penis called the *corpus cavernosum,* which consists of arteries, veins, and muscle tissue. Under a relaxed, sexually stimulated state, blood pours into this sponge-like structure unimpeded and becomes trapped, resulting in an erection.

Western-trained physicians in China have performed study after study with cordyceps in the treatment of male impotence. In one study, the Department of Neurology at Hua Shan Hospital in Shanghai tested the mycelium product in 286 impotent men. After taking one gram of cordyceps three times a day for forty days, 183 patients reported some improvement in sexual functioning. At the end of another forty days, almost half of the men reported that their sex lives had been partially or completely restored.

When word got out, others wanted to begin their own trials. The Shanghai Institute of Endocrinology elected to try two 20-day courses of cordyceps in fifty impotent men. After they had completed both courses of the mycelium, thirteen patients reported that they had been able to resume sexual activity. Another twelve subjects indicated that they were experiencing sexual sensations and were now able to have erections.

The Department of Neurosurgery at the Medical School of Suchou also recruited fifty impotent patients. They ran before-and-after tests on the patients for levels of the male sex hormone *metabolites 17-ketosteroid,* which are reported to be low in impotent men. Researchers found that levels of the sex hormone rose in the men who took cordyceps mycelium. In fact, thirty-two patients reported that their conditions had improved significantly. The doctors concluded that cordyceps cures erectile dysfunction in the majority of men.

This study also suggests that cordyceps has other benefits. Lower back pain, or *lumbago,* generally improved in the patients who took cordyceps. In addition, they experienced less weakness of the lower limbs; fewer incidences of insomnia, dizziness, and vertigo; and improvements in mental state. And the plasma levels of sex hormones—testosterone, cortisol, and estradiol—increased to normal levels.

CONCLUSION

It seems that the centuries-old use of cordyceps as a medicine to help men with erectile dysfunction has been overlooked by the pharmaceutical industry in the West. Of course, more clinical tests are needed, but every study to date has concluded that cordyceps can be of great value to men suffering from erectile dysfunction. This was true whether the source of the problem was physical, mental, or emotional.

CHAPTER 6

CORDYCEPS AND KIDNEY DISEASE

The kidneys are among the body's most complex organs. When they fail, all other organs are affected. Kidney disease is the eighth leading cause of death in the United States among people age sixty-five to seventy-four; and the cost of treating advanced kidney disease is at least 11 billion dollars a year. There is encouraging news, though, that cordyceps may help reduce that cost in several ways. Clinical research has shown that cordyceps improves the condition of patients with chronic kidney failure and decreases kidney toxicity caused by antibiotics used to treat kidney disease. Furthermore, cordyceps reduces the toxicity of powerful medications that are given to prevent organ rejection in kidney transplant patients.

VIEWS OF THE KIDNEYS

Doctors of traditional Chinese and Western medicine agree that healthy kidneys are essential for the body's good health and well-being. The difference in their views is reflected in the Chinese belief that the jing is stored in the kidneys. You may recall from the discussion in Chapter 5 that the jing is responsible for the flow of Qi, or life force, throughout the body.

Traditional Chinese Medicine's View of the Kidneys

Traditional Chinese medicine holds the view that all organs of the body are completely dependent upon the kidneys for their life activity. For that reason, TCM doctors say that the kidneys are the "root of life." They also believe that the kidneys are responsible for the integrity of the bones, and in particular, for marrow production. Kidneys that are low in jing are believed to be the cause of brittle bones, a stiff spine, weakness in the knees and legs, and hair loss. In TCM, the kidneys are also closely associated with the ears, and hearing problems are routinely treated with herbs specific for the kidneys.

When the yang energy of the kidneys is exhausted, the body appears swollen, the lower part of the back feels heavy and sore, there is little urine, and the limbs are sensitive to the cold. According to TCM, cordyceps can benefit patients with these symptoms.

Traditional Western Medicine's View of the Kidneys

In Western medicine, we see the kidneys from a similar perspective. The kidneys regulate fluid balance in the body, which of course affects all the organs and systems of the body. In addition, we know that damage to the kidneys can lead to bone disorders such as osteoporosis and osteosclerosis. And, indeed, there is a link between the ears and the kidneys, which can be seen in cases of hearing loss resulting from an immunological kidney disorder known as Berger's disease. We will discuss Berger's disease in detail later in the chapter. The following list summarizes the functions of the kidneys.

❑ The kidneys maintain:

- Water balance

- Acid-base balance

- Electrolyte balance

- Hemoglobin and red blood cells

- Phosphorus and calcium balance

❑ The kidneys filter and reabsorb:

- Potassium

- Salt

- Magnesium

- Phosphate

❑ The kidneys synthesize:

- *Autocoids,* which are chemicals that act like local hormones or messengers between one cell and another (e.g., prostaglandins, kinins, renins)

- Active hormones (e.g., *erythropoietin,* a hormone secreted by the kidneys that makes bone marrow cells stimulate the production of red blood cells)[1]

KIDNEY DISEASES

In traditional Chinese medicine, cordyceps is prescribed mainly as a tonic for the kidneys. In fact, the mushroom has been prescribed as a kidney-strengthening herbal medicine for hundreds of years, but until recently few Western doctors knew anything about it.

In China, cordyceps is the main ingredient in an herbal formula used for the treatment of chronic kidney failure and other kidney diseases. Yet many doctors prescribe cordyceps without using it with other herbs or drugs. Extensive research has been conducted in China and, more recently, in the West, that confirms the effectiveness of cordyceps in treating some kidney diseases. Let's look at three of these disorders: chronic renal failure, acute kidney failure, and Berger's disease.

Chronic Renal (Kidney) Failure

Chronic renal failure, or CRF, is a progressive kidney disease that can be caused by a number of other diseases. CRF patients are not able to eliminate excess salt and water from their bodies, and this causes extensive damage to all systems and organs of the body. Most cases result from diabetes, high blood pressure, and obstructions in the urinary tract. Atherosclerosis, cardiac arrest, depression, excess body weight, and a number of other disorders can also cause the disease. The prognosis for patients with CRF is not good.

The conventional treatment of chronic renal failure includes dialysis and medications such as prednisone, which prevent the immune system from attacking the kidneys. The problem is that some medications produce side effects such as retarded growth in children, osteoporosis, and damage to the nervous system. In fact, no therapy has proven to be beneficial beyond giving temporary relief from CRF, and researchers are constantly looking for treatment alternatives. In many cases of chronic renal failure, the only solution is a kidney transplant.

Cordyceps and CRF

Researchers in China report that cordyceps can help patients with chronic renal failure. A clinical study of thirty-seven CRF patients treated with a daily dosage of 5 grams of cordyceps for thirty days found significant improvements. Compared with the results of pre-treatment tests, red blood cell and hemoglobin counts were greatly increased. The most improvement was shown in a *creatinine clearance test*, which measures the kidney-filtration rate in terms of a waste product called *serum creatinine.* Tests showed an improvement rate of about 39 percent. In addition, there was a 34-percent decrease in *blood urea nitrogen,* or BUN. A high level of BUN is a major indicator of kidney disease, heart failure, dehydration, intestinal bleeding, muscle degeneration, diabetic acidosis, and an increased breakdown of protein. The test subjects also showed increased levels of SOD, one of the body's free-radical scavengers (see Chapter 3). And their arterial blood pressure had dropped by an average of 15 percent. Equally important was the 63-percent drop in proteins found in their urine, which is one of the strongest indicators of an overall correction of kidney function.

In a similar study of thirty CRF patients, researchers noted improvements in the rate of *lymphocyte transformation.* A low rate indicates poor immune function and is typically seen in chemotherapy patients and in people suffering from AIDS, lymphoma, burns, and malnutrition.

Improvements in T-lymphocyte cells were witnessed in another clinical study of fifty-one CRF patients who had been treated with cordyceps for ten months. The per formance of these cells—also called T-helper cells because they help other immune cells protect the body—improved by about 13 percent. The researchers conducting the study found a correlation between improvements in immune cells and improvements in kidney function. Cordyceps appeared to have restored some balance to the immune system. What's more, there was a 25-percent improvement in BUN levels. Hemoglobin counts rose by 18 percent, and rates of creatinine clearance increased by over 30 percent.

Acute Kidney Failure

Acute kidney failure is distinguished from chronic renal failure in that its onset causes rapid deterioration of the kidneys, which impairs their ability to clear toxic substances from the blood. As a result, waste products such as urea accumulate in the blood. Treatment options depend a great deal on whether or not the patient has experienced failure of other organs of the body. If it is treated before it damages the other organs, acute kidney failure has a 90-percent cure rate. However, in extreme cases, dialysis may be necessary.

Cordyceps and Acute Kidney Failure

Cordyceps can relieve acute kidney failure brought on by an adverse reaction to antibiotics such as *aminoglycosides.* Studies have shown that cordyceps has significant kidney-protective effects against *gentamicin* and a related aminoglycoside known as *kanamycin.* In a controlled study of patients who had developed a condition called *gentamicin kidney toxicity,* which is an adverse reaction to the aminoglycoside gentamicin, half the patients were given an extract of the cultured mycelium of cordyceps while still taking gentamicin. The control group continued to receive the gentamicin and additional drugs to neutralize its toxicity. By the sixth day, 89 percent of the cordyceps group had made a complete clinical recovery from the toxicity of gentamicin. In comparison, only 45 percent of the control group recovered.

Berger's Disease

Berger's disease is the most common form of a kidney disease called *glomerulonephritis,* which damages the basic filtering units of the kidneys. Known for its slow but relentless progression, Berger's disease is marked with constant deposits in the kidneys of a class of antibodies known as *immunoglobulin A* (IgA). The persistence of these deposits leads to the appearance of various kidney lesions in what amounts to a constant cycle of deposits, inflammations, and lesions. Despite recent research, the cause of Berger's disease and its cure remain unknown.

Berger's disease is named after the Parisian pathologist who described it in 1968. It mainly affects men in their twenties and thirties. In about one-third of cases, it can take up to twenty-five years to develop. In other cases, however, onset can be swift. Signs associated with the disease include high blood pressure, a decrease in kidney function, and the presence of blood and high amounts of protein in the urine. It's estimated that 10 to 40 percent of Berger's disease patients will eventually develop end-stage kidney disease. When this happens, patients require a kidney transplant in order to survive. Insufficient knowledge and the absence of clinically effective treatments have left many physicians undecided about whether or not to bother treating the disease. Why? Because treatments for Berger's disease—concentrated fish oil, ACE inhibitors, blood thinners, and immunosuppressants such as azathioprine and corticosteroids—have produced conflicting or even toxic results from one trial to the next. Some appear to slow the progression of Berger's disease and others show no great benefit at all. But because no effective treatments have been discovered, doctors still perform clinical tests with these substances to see which works best. On the bright side, about 12 percent of patients experience complete remission from the disease after eight years. Still, no one knows why.

Cordyceps and Berger's Disease

In recent years, promising results with cordyceps, vitamin E, and Chinese medicinal herbs have begun to attract the attention of kidney specialists. Some Western-trained doctors have even expressed an interest in treating kidney diseases with herbal medicines. With nothing to stop Berger's disease from progressing, research continues to focus on the immune system for clues to stop or slow its course.

A specialist in the treatment of kidney diseases at Veterans General Hospital in Taipei, Taiwan, Dr. Ching-Yuan Lin seems to have been the first to demonstrate that cordyceps may be a valuable aid in the treatment of Berger's disease. Dr. Lin developed a method of extracting bioactive agents from natural products such as cordyceps, and he uses them to suppress the cells that contribute to Berger's disease. His method became a patented invention for extracting an element from cordyceps that seems to alleviate the symptoms of Berger's disease and prevent the disease from progressing to a more severe stage.

KIDNEY TRANSPLANTS

With the advent of kidney transplantation in the 1970s, the way was opened to transplant other vital organs, which has saved countless lives. The majority of patients who require kidney transplants suffer from diabetes mellitus with kidney failure, hypertension with advanced stage kidney disease, and patients with glomerulonephritis, an inflammation of the small blood vessels in the urine filters of the kidneys.

Cordyceps and Kidney Transplants

Laboratory tests on cordyceps indicate that it help to counteract the toxic side effects of gentamicin, and it provides protection against the toxicity of *cyclosporine,* one of the drugs used to prevent the immune system from rejecting newly transplanted organs. Cyclosporine is a very useful immunosuppressant that has saved many lives. But because of its deleterious effect on the kidneys, the drug presents a difficult problem for transplant patients who rely on it for survival. By constricting blood vessels and causing damage to kidney cells, cyclosporine can induce acute kidney failure. It can also cause diabetes mellitus, hypertension, and cancer, and it can make patients susceptible to infections.

In one clinical study of cordyceps, researchers selected seven kidney-transplant patients who were taking the conventional cocktail of anti-rejection agents—azathioprine, cyclosporine, and prednisone. All the subjects had developed low levels of infection-fighting white blood cells and other symptoms of organ rejection. Cordyceps was administered as a replacement for the toxic azathioprine. Researchers determined that cordyceps had caused no inhibition of the leukocytes. In fact, their levels returned to normal, thereby allowing the immune system to combat infections.

A larger placebo-controlled clinical study of cordyceps in kidney-transplant patients was conducted by the Department of Clinical Pharmacology of Nanfang Hospital and Taizhou Medical School in China. The purpose of the trial was to test the ability of cordyceps to protect the kidneys from cyclosporine toxicity. Sixty-nine stable kidney-transplant patients were randomly assigned to one of two groups. One group of thirty-nine patients received a placebo. All the patients received cyclosporine, and throughout the fifteen-day trial, they were monitored for signs of kidney toxicity. Researchers found less kidney toxicity in the cordyceps group. In addition, the study showed that the longer patients took the mushroom powder, the less toxicity there was. Based on their findings and those of other researchers in China, the doctors who conducted the trial now recommend cordyceps for kidney-transplant patients on cyclosporine.

CONCLUSION

I found physicians at the Longhua Hospital in Shanghai who had used cordyceps to treat around 40,000 cases of kidney disease. I came away with the impression that the use of cordyceps in kidney disease had barely been tapped in the rest of the world.

Dr. Mariana Markell is a kidney specialist at the Health Science Center of the State University of New York who prescribes herbs to treat patients with kidney disease. She cautions that herbs, which can affect a patient's regular medications, should only be taken with the utmost care and with the knowledge and cooperation of the attending physician. She adds that although herbal medicines might allow patients to cut down on their pharmaceuticals, this precaution is especially warranted in treating diabetics. Extra care must also be taken when treating patients undergoing kidney dialysis and patients who have had kidney transplants.

Medicinal plants hold enormous promise in the treatment of kidney disease, and there are many good reasons to believe that cordyceps is a tonic for the kidneys par excellence. Nevertheless, studies concerning cordyceps and kidney disease are only beginning in the West. Like all medicinal substances, cordyceps must be used with a great deal of care when treating serious cases. Although the mushroom may be one of the best studied "kidney herbs" when it comes to treating particular kinds of kidney disease, there is still a great deal that we don't know.

CHAPTER 7

CORDYCEPS AND THE RESPIRATORY SYSTEM

The old Chinese texts state that cordyceps goes to the meridians of the kidneys and lungs. For centuries, cordyceps has been the medicine of choice in TCM for treating respiratory diseases. During the twentieth century, doctors in China have prescribed cordyceps for chronic bronchitis, asthma, pulmonary and congestive heart diseases, and tuberculosis. Cordyceps is said to stop continual coughing, reduce phlegm, and cure illnesses of the diaphragm. In its simplest use for the lungs, cordyceps is taken to relieve bronchial inflammation and acts as an expectorant. Laboratory studies support the use of cordyceps for the treatment of respiratory diseases. For example, we now know that the extract of the cultured mycelium inhibits contractions in the trachea, indicating that cordyceps increases the flow of air in the airways.

VIEWS OF THE RESPIRATORY SYSTEM

In traditional Chinese medicine, the lungs are said to rule the Qi, which is associated with the element of air. When the lungs are in a healthy state, the Qi flows unimpeded into and out of the lungs. But if the current of Qi is ob-structed or becomes impaired in some way, it can bring about a deficiency in the body's life force.

In Western terms, the respiratory system includes the lungs, the bronchi, the tonsils, the larynx, and all airways. It is responsible for the exchange of carbon dioxide and oxygen between a living organism and the environment. If one of the respiratory organs doesn't function properly, damage to the body can range from minor to severe. The following sections will examine some common respiratory problems and the use of cordyceps in alleviating them.

RESPIRATORY DISEASES

The incidence of lung and lung-related disorders is grow-ing worldwide. These include asthma and occupational diseases such as chronic bronchitis and black lung. Other diseases of the lung are the result of disorders of the air-ways such as chronic obstructive pulmonary disease. One of the benefits of cordyceps in the treatment of lung dis-eases may be that it causes increased activity of the body's own antioxidant, *superoxide dismutase,* or SOD. In the fol-lowing sections, we will examine some disorders of the lungs and pulmonary tract and the role of cordyceps in their treatment.

Chronic Bronchitis

Chronic bronchitis affects as many as 25 percent of adults. The incidence of chronic bronchitis is particularly high in people who work in dusty environments, and it more com-monly strikes people over the age of forty. The chronic coughing in bronchitis is the result of an accumulation of lung secretions.

I know that many people think bronchitis is a tempo-rary ailment brought on by a bad cold. But bronchitis can get much more serious. It can develop into chronic bronchitis, a condition in which the patient has a lower resistance to bronchial infections and a productive, or sputum-producing, cough every day for three or more months.

Cigarette smoking has been identified as a main cause of bronchitis, but that doesn't explain why roughly half of smokers don't develop chronic bronchitis or, for that matter, why only 10 to 15 percent of smokers suffer from chronically limited airflow. In an effort to understand these exceptions, researchers from two Italian universities recently examined bronchial biopsy specimens from chronic bronchitis patients. Smokers with chronic bronchitis whose airflow was limited showed significantly greater numbers of macrophages and T lymphocytes than smokers with chronic bronchitis whose airflow was not limited. These differences, which may underlie chronic airway obstruction, are probably related to the hyper-responsiveness of the immune system seen in chronic bronchitis. A study by the National Heart and Lung Institute in London found indications of a relationship between increased airflow obstruction and greater numbers of T lymphocytes and macrophages. Researchers also found associations between impaired lung function and inflammatory cells.

Cordyceps and Chronic Bronchitis

What do these findings tell us about cordyceps? Simply put, they hint at the possibility that cordyceps acts on an immunological level in treating bronchitis. It's possible that by calming the hyper-responses of the respiratory immune system, which lead to inflammation and reduced airflow, cordyceps earned a reputation in traditional Chinese medicine as an aid in relieving problems of the lungs, continual coughing, and the buildup of phlegm.

Chinese researchers have conducted numerous clinical trials of cordyceps in the treatment of chronic bronchitis.

In one study, patients between the ages of fifty-five and sixty were randomly divided into two groups. All had been suffering from chronic bronchitis for about twelve years. The twenty-seven patients in the study group received 3 grams of cordyceps three times a day for four weeks. The control group received a similar amount of a berry extract called *Oleum Viticis negundo*, which is commonly used in China to treat coughs, colds, wheezing, and bronchitis. At the end of the study, twenty-one patients in the cordyceps group found relief from their symptoms, whereas only eight patients in the control group felt any improvement.

A second one-month trial with thirty-five patients was completed the following year. Jiangxi Medical College reported that cordyceps had helped as many as 90 percent of the patients, or eighteen of the twenty people in the study group. This compared to a mere 20-percent improvement rate in the control group. Medical examinations showed a significant increase in pulmonary function in the cordyceps group. Patients experienced fewer bronchial spasms, coughing spells, and incidences of airway resistance. There were also significant increases in maximum breathing capacity and *forced expiratory volume*, or FEV1, tests, which measure the amount of air that a patient can expel in one second. In this instance, the cordyceps patients showed about 40 percent more capacity than did patients in the control group.

An exploratory survey in 1995 marked a revival of interest in cordyceps for the treatment of respiratory illnesses. Researchers at the Department of Pulmonary Medicine in Jiang-Su Provincial Hospital reported preliminary findings in 100 respiratory disease patients, the majority of whom had chronic bronchitis complicated with pulmonary heart disease or emphysema. Following two weeks of treatment with cordyceps, they found that patients caught fewer colds, showed improved expectoration and cough, and had fewer asthmatic symptoms. In addition, patients reported relief from night sweats, and their appetites began to return. Since the Jiang-Su survey showed that 92 percent of patients taking cordyceps improved in one or more of these functions, it is logical to suppose that cordyceps could help patients with other respiratory diseases.

Chronic Obstructive Pulmonary Disease (COPD)

Chronic obstructive pulmonary disease refers to obstruction of the air passages caused by disorders such as emphysema and bronchitis. In patients with hyperactive airways, exposure to irritants can cause smooth-muscle constriction, or *bronchospasm,* and excess production of mucus and swelling of the bronchial walls. When these spasms become recurrent, the condition becomes *asthmatic bronchitis.* In chronic asthmatic bronchitis, patients are plagued with bronchospasms, cough all the time, and suffer from airway obstruction. Because these symptoms also occur in emphysema, the term *chronic obstructive pulmonary disease,* or COPD, is often used to include the whole group of respiratory diseases associated with bronchial obstruction.

Patients with COPD usually suffer from some other chronic health problem. Of the 15 million people in the United States with COPD, 12.5 million have some form of chronic bronchitis. Others suffer from problems such as rheumatism, hypertension, circulatory and heart ailments, and prostate disorders.

In traditional Western medicine, COPD is treated with bronchodilators that allow the airways to ventilate more freely. The drugs administered as bronchodilators are primarily beta-agonists and anticholinergics. Side effects from beta-agonists can include muscle tremors, changes in blood pressure, headaches, and restlessness. Oxygen inhalation may provide relief of symptoms in more advanced cases. There is no known cure for COPD.

Cordyceps and COPD

Cordyceps has proven to be effective in at least one formal study of people suffering from COPD. The study group included eleven women and twenty-four men, aged fifty-six to seventy-nine. All had been hospitalized after acute onset of symptoms of emphysema with persistent cough, excessive production of phlegm, pulmonary infections, gasping, and *hypoxia,* or poor tissue supply of oxygen. Ten of the patients were suffering from heart failure and various pulmonary heart diseases. A few of the patients were being treated with cardiotonic drugs, and all were being treated with antibiotics, expectorants, and anti-asthmatic medications. Once their conditions had stabilized, they were given 330 milligrams of cordyceps three times a day. After twenty-one days, their levels of the antioxidant SOD showed a highly significant 35.7 percent increase. The increase indicated that tissue repair and protective mechanisms had gone into higher gear. By the end of the study, all the patients showed a marked improvement in pulmonary signs of COPD, appetite, and general physical problems including coughing, gasping, and the production of phlegm.

Asthma

Asthma is defined as a chronic inflammatory disorder of the airways, which results in their narrowing. An allergic reaction to dust and pollen, smoke, pollutants, and other stimuli may cause the narrowing. In the United States, 5 percent of the population suffers from asthma. There is no cure for the disorder. The best anyone can hope for is symptom control.

The inflammatory nature of asthma is seen in recurring spells of wheezing, cough, tightness in the chest, and breathlessness. The disorder is brought about by various cells of the immune system that appear to have gone into overdrive and remain in a chronically activated state. Certain commonly used drugs, such as aspirin and ibuprofen, can also exacerbate the symptoms of asthma.

Western treatment of asthma consists of *beta-adrenergic receptor agonists,* which are bronchodilators that widen the airways, and anti-inflammatory drugs such as inhaled corticosteroids. In some extreme cases, oxygen must be given along with the bronchodilators. Asthma attacks can be life-threatening events. The choice of drugs and the frequency of their administration are based on the severity of symptoms, but the most effective agents to date are anti-inflammatories such as inhaled corticosteroids.

Cordyceps and Asthma

My colleagues in China tell me that they commonly prescribe cordyceps for the treatment of asthma. In at least one clinical study of cordyceps arranged by Beijing Medical University, cordyceps proved to be beneficial to asthma patients. Fifty asthma patients ranging in age from seventeen to sixty-five were recruited for the study. All had previously been treated unsuccessfully with antibiotics and other commonly prescribed Western medications. The patients were examined to rule out any other diseases; in addition, all tested poor (20 percent) for FEV1. Thirty-two subjects assigned to the cordyceps group received 3 grams of cordyceps or 10 milligrams of the antihistamine *astemizole* for ten days. Researchers reported that the total effective rate for the cordyceps group was 81.3 percent. This means that FEV1 scores improved in ten patients, and another sixteen patients had increased their FEV1 scores by 20 percent. Subjects in the antihistamine group showed a total effective rate of 61.1 percent. Only six of the patients showed full relief from cough and chest oppression and had increased FEV1 scores. Treatment was not at all effective in seven patients. For patients in the cordyceps group, it took an average of only five days to improve; but it took nine days for cough to subside for those in the antihistamine group. The only side effect was heartburn in two patients, which was quickly remedied when they took their medications following meals instead of before.

CONCLUSION

For the growing numbers of people affected by diseases of the lungs and airways, there is no doubt that cordyceps is a valuable element in the line of defense. Although clinical studies in the West are still limited, the fact is that doctors of TCM have used cordyceps in the successful treatment of lung-related disorders since ancient times. It is not without reason that cordyceps is famous for nourishing the lungs.

CHAPTER 8

CORDYCEPS AND THE IMMUNE SYSTEM

From a medical standpoint, cordyceps is the most investigated medicinal mushroom. As more accurate assessments accrue from more definitive studies, the strides retold here will fade into footnotes. Advances in medical technology will only allow the level of research into cordyceps to increase. There are several areas of research that might give us an idea of where these studies will lead, and they all concern the immune system.

An increasing amount of cordyceps research suggests that it acts as an *immunoregulator*. This means that cordyceps increases the activity of select immune system cells when their activity is too low, and decreases activities of immune system cells when they are too high. So far, the label of immunoregulator is theoretical. This label describes any substance that can quiet or activate the immune system depending on circumstances.

THE FUNCTION OF THE IMMUNE SYSTEM

The job of the immune system is to defend the body against invasion by foreign cells or substances. It does this by recognizing invading cells or bodies, engaging its forces, and attacking the invaders. The network of cells that constitute the immune system extends to practically every part of the body. Collectively, immune cells form a protective barrier against millions of disease-causing organisms and cell-damaging chemicals. There are two parts to the immune system—one part produces antibodies and the other produces immunity via the cells. When the immune system functions in a balanced way, we are relatively healthy. But when it is less than efficient, the body becomes more susceptible to disease.

The lymphocytes are among the main cells of the immune system. About one percent of them circulate in the bloodstream, and the rest circulate in specialized organs such as the thymus gland, lymph nodes, and spleen. Lymphocytes migrate to the bloodstream and are distributed throughout the body to check for contaminants and infections.

DISEASES OF THE IMMUNE SYSTEM

The immune system, like any other system of the body, is susceptible to a number of diseases. Diseases of the immune system are called *immune disorders*, and they include diabetes, lupus, AIDS, and cancer, all of which have been studied in connection with cordyceps. If it can be demonstrated that cordyceps is effective in helping patients suffering from these diseases, it will certainly have positive implications for other immune disorders.

Diabetes

Diabetes is an immune-system disorder in which blood sugar levels are abnormally high, either because the body doesn't produce insulin or because the body isn't able to use insulin effectively. Left untreated, it can be life threatening. The immunological affront in diabetes is now fairly well known. The process is believed to start out from factors in the host's environment, which may be chemicals, viruses, poor nutrition, or a combination of factors. Whatever the factors, they cause diabetes by triggering immune-system cells that target beta cells in the pancreas, the very cells that produce insulin. Once that happens, a message goes out to every post in the immune system to capture these beta cells, dead or alive. Now you have an autoimmune reaction. Macrophages, which operate by engulfing and destroying foreign cells, are only too eager to oblige. The trouble is, they can't keep their mouths shut, and soon trigger-happy helper T cells also want to get into the act. The helper T cells send recruitment notices, or *cytokines*, to associates who arrange to make life miserable for the beta cells. Meanwhile, the macrophages have become all fired up, and with guns loaded, go after the beta cells on their own. The result is that the body has no way of regulating the buildup of sugar in the bloodstream that would normally be regulated by the beta cells.

Cordyceps and Diabetes

Cordyceps entered the milieu of diabetes research in 1993. University laboratories in China and Japan reported significant sugar-lowering, or hypoglycemic, effects from extracts of the cultured mycelium of cordyceps, and from sugars isolated from the mycelium known as *mannans*, or *polysaccharides*. In 1995, a group of researchers in China arranged a clinical study of forty-two diabetics. Patients received the mycelium powder as part of a formula of herbal medicines, the ingredients of which the researchers chose not to divulge. The trial ran for thirty days with a test group of twenty patients taking cordyceps plus the mysterious herbal formula, and a control group of twenty-two patients taking only the herbal formula. Patients in the control group showed symptomatic improvements in

54.5 percent of cases, with no improvements in any of the remaining 45.5 percent. Those in the cordyceps group improved in 95 percent of cases, or all but one patient. At the end of the treatment period, researchers ran tests for *proteinuria,* which is the urinary excretion of proteins. Proteinuria is a general indicator of disease advancement, and it can indicate the development of secondary complications in diabetes such as kidney disease, liver disease, or heart disease. The rate of proteinuria had increased by 16.7 percent in the control group, whereas only half the patients in the cordyceps group showed any proteinuria.

The research on cordyceps in diabetes is still very new, and we don't know specifically how diabetics are helped by the mushroom. It seems, however, that cordyceps may calm or quiet the cells of the immune system involved in diabetes. Although more testing is needed, those studies that have been conducted are very promising.

Lupus

Lupus is another immune-complex disease for which effective treatments are still lacking and the cause is unknown. Lupus is an autoimmune disease known as *systemic lupus erythematosus,* or SLE. Although lupus can strike at any age, most cases occur in people between sixteen and fifty-five. The disorder mostly affects Asian women during their childbearing years and also appears among blacks in the Caribbean. Its name derives from the appearance of a red patch on the forehead that resembles a V-shape, like the dark patch on the forehead of a wolf (*L. lupus*). The symptoms are variable and appear in combinations of fatigue, rashes, persistent proteinuria, inflammation of the fluid membrane surrounding the lungs, arthritis, anemia, seizures, oral ulcers, and low white blood cell counts. Many lupus patients have signs of fatigue, anxiety, or depression. The disease is treated with immunosuppressants, steroids, nonsteroidal anti-inflammatory drugs, and antimalarials for the muscle pains, rashes, and fever.

Cordyceps and Lupus

Researchers at the Kaohsiung Medical College in Taiwan have been treating lupus patients with various Chinese herbs to find alternatives to the available drugs and their side effects, which include bone disorders, immune-system suppression, cataracts, and suppression of the adrenal glands. Five herbs were found that improve the production of the immune-system messenger of *interleukin-2*, which some authorities believe are a main feature of the disease. The herbs in question are cordyceps, *Angelica sinensis* or dong quai, *Ligustrum lucidum*, *Codonopsis pilosula*, and *Atractylodes ovata*. These five herbs were tested in 144 mice that had developed lupus naturally. Laboratory tests indicated that cordyceps had significantly lengthened their life span and significantly inhibited the production of antibodies to their own DNA, which are known as *anti-double-stranded DNA*, or dsDNA. After six months, 87.5 percent of the cordyceps group tested negative for dsDNA. And after eight months, 75 percent of the mice that were being given the extract of cordyceps were still alive.

AIDS

Although we don't know precisely how long *acquired immunodeficiency syndrome,* better known as AIDS, has been around, it was first diagnosed in the early 1980s. AIDS is caused by an infection called *human immunodeficiency virus,* or HIV, which involves the progressive destruction of various white blood cells known as *lymphocytes.*

Cordyceps and AIDS

Wild cordyceps was known to the so-called AIDS underground in the United States and Europe during the late 1980s. People were taking the mushroom in the hope of raising their helper T-cell levels. But whether it helped anyone over the long-term is anyone's guess. Several years ago, it was rumored that AIDS patients in Tanzania were taking cordyceps. But until 1995, I had no idea that another rumor—one about a secret African herbal formula that caused HIV symptoms to disappear—had anything to do with cordyceps and its use in traditional Chinese medicine.

In 1995, the *Chinese Medical Journal* published a report on the long-term use of herbal formulas that seemed to be making a profound difference in HIV patients. The formulas were indeed a secret. Few people outside the group of researchers—four doctors from the Academy of Traditional Chinese Medicine of China in Beijing and three from the Muhimbili Medical Center in Tanzania—knew exactly what ingredients went into them. Finally, doctors at the Beijing International Conference of Traditional Medicine announced that they had given six different Chinese herbal formulas to 158 HIV-positive patients in Tanzania. Among the chief ingredients in all their formulas were cordyceps, licorice root, *Astragalus,* and *huang qin,* an herb often used in traditional Chinese medicine to treat fevers. Two years later, they reported that HIV symptoms seemed to have disappeared in eight patients ages twenty to forty-eight. When doctors double-checked, they learned that patients' symptoms were in fact fluctuating from negative to positive and back again. For most of the test subjects, symptoms and signs of AIDS had disappeared after there were improvements in their T-cell counts. Of course, it would take many more studies to determine whether or not these formulas work. At the very least, the doctors hope that their formulas may prolong the time between a diagnosis of HIV and the onset of AIDS.

Cancer

Cancer is a complex immune-associated disease that can affect any organ or system of the body. It is caused by uncontrolled cell growth resulting from a genetic defect or cellular damage due to radiation or toxins in the environment. Although many advances have been made in the field of cancer research, there is still much to be done. Unfortunately, treatments such as radiation and chemotherapy can be as debilitating to the patient as the cancer itself. But recent research indicates that traditional therapy when used in combination with alternative therapies may help cancer patients.

Cordyceps and Cancer

Since 1979, reports from China have suggested that cordyceps may benefit cancer patients. Several cases of lung carcinoma treated with cordyceps were reported to have shown significant improvements. Later, a clinical study sought to learn about the immunological effect of cordyceps in patients with advanced cancers, such as those of the breast, liver, gastrointestinal tract, lymph glands, pancreas, lungs, smooth muscles, prostate, cervix, and vagina. Since none of the patients was expected to live more than two months, all drugs that would affect the immune system were stopped while researchers checked immune system functions. The patients continued to receive chemotherapy in addition to a traditional herbal formula to make them more comfortable. The patients, who ranged in age from twenty-one to seventy, were randomly assigned to two groups. The thirty-six subjects in the test group received 330 milligrams of cordyceps three times a day for sixty days. After the treatment ended, there were some obvious differences between patients in the test group and those in the control group, who had not taken cordyceps.

An increase was found in T lymphocytes, lymphocyte reproduction, and surface proteins on T lymphocytes in every patient in the cordyceps group, but there was no such progress in the control group. The most interesting results are reflected in the patients' symptoms, which are summarized in Table 8.1. The group on the TCM formula with conventional chemotherapy also showed improved symptoms, although not nearly as much as when cordyceps was part of the therapy.

**Table 8.1. Symptom Improvements in Advanced
Stage Cancer Patients**

	TCM + Chemotherapy + Cordyceps	TCM + Chemotherapy
Fever	89% or 32/36 patients	85% or 17/20 patients
Anorexia	83% or 30/36 patients	25% or 5/20 patients
Vomiting	56% or 20/36 patients	40% or 8/20 patients
Fatigue	81% or 29/36 patients	30% or 6/20 patients
Pain	50% or 18/36 patients	45% or 9/20 patients
Overall Improvement	72% or 27/36 patients	45% or 16/36 patients

Adapted from D.H. Zhou and L.Z Lin, 1995

Researchers conducted another study of cordyceps in advanced-stage lung cancer patients who were about to undergo chemotherapy and radiation treatments. Twenty-five of the thirty-nine patients who didn't receive cordyceps completed their therapies, and nineteen of the twenty patients taking cordyceps completed their therapies. Following chemotherapy and radiation treatments, blood counts were normal in about 60 percent of control-group patients. In comparison, blood counts were normal in about 85 percent of cordyceps patients. This indicates that cordyceps can improve patients' tolerance to chemotherapy and radiation, and that it decreases the toxic effects of these treatments on bone marrow. The results also suggest that patients on cordyceps may have a better chance of completing cancer therapy, which may improve their chances of survival.

A similar study of lung cancer patients who were receiving chemotherapy and TCM herbal formulas recorded the changes effected by the addition of cordyceps. The sizes of tumors were partially reduced in twenty-three of the fifty patients, and the majority showed improvements in subjective symptoms such as malaise, pain, and fatigue.

Cordyceps was also tested in a group of fifty lung-cancer patients. For over twenty months, the patients received chemotherapy and radiation in addition to cordyceps and herbal formulas, which were administered and formulated according to individual patient needs. Researchers reported subjective symptom improvements in almost every patient and tumors had decreased in size in nearly half the patients. However, no changes of any significance were found in immune cell counts. Table 8.2 summarizes the changes in the size of the patients' tumors.

Table 8.2. Changes in Lung Cancer Patients Treated with Cordyceps, TCM Herbs, and Conventional Therapies

Change	Number of Patients
Symptoms improved by 68%–100%	50
Tumor size increased	1
Tumor size reduced by 50% or more	6
Tumor size reduced by 25%, but less than 50%	15
Tumor size reduced by less than 25% or not at all	9
Tumor disappeared completely	2

Adapted from R.J. Yan et al, 1992

Researchers have yet to figure out exactly how cordyceps worked to improve the condition of these cancer patients. Laboratory tests have shown that cordyceps has anti-immunosuppressive and immunopotentiating influences. This means that cordyceps seems to have increased the responsiveness of the immune system and counteracted the immune system-suppressing effects of cancer. Furthermore, cordyceps has shown bone marrow-protective and antileukemic activities. Other tests have demonstrated that cordyceps can inhibit the growth of a wide range of tumors such as lymphomas, melanomas, and sarcomas. Cordyceps can also counteract the immunosuppressing effects of agents such as cortisone, prednisolone, and others.

During the 1980s, studies demonstrated that cordyceps enhanced the effects of some anticancer drugs against tumors. It wasn't clear at first whether or not this had resulted from increased immunological activity. Then in 1993, a report published by Norman Bethune University announced that cordyceps inhibits the growth of carcinoma cells in the larynx. The following year, the National Research Institute of Chinese Medicine and Dr. C.Y. Lin, who had researched the treatment of Berger's disease with cordyceps, discovered two elements in wild cordyceps that inhibit the growth of tumors. When they exposed tumor cells to these inhibitors, there was a significant decrease in the growth rates of five different cancer cells: one was a type of red blood leukemia cell; another was a type of kidney tumor cell; and the others were lung cancer cells and skin tumor cells. But the odd thing was that they did not show the cell-destructive action one might expect. Instead, they acted by inhibiting the production of DNA in the tumor cells, which effectively stopped the cells from growing.

While I believe that cordyceps has potential as an extremely good immunoregulator, the mystery remains as to how it manages to act as needed and why it seems to act in an immunoregulatory fashion at all. Perhaps the answers will come sooner than we think.

In 1994, immunologists in China reported that immune cells known as natural-killer cells taken from patients with leukemia at the stage of remission were significantly inhibited when exposed to a water extract of wild cordyceps. Yet, the natural-killer cells taken from leukemia patients still in the active stage of leukemia were significantly stimulated by the same amount of cordyceps.

CONCLUSION

In summary, cordyceps appears to be selective in the way it acts on immune cells. Treatment with cordyceps has been shown to boost sluggish immune systems, as well as to calm those that are overly active. Definitive answers about the bi-directional immune activity of cordyceps, however, are not yet forthcoming. There is no consensus even among the most knowledgeable researchers. This is because results depend on many factors such as test procedures, dosage, type of preparations, state of the patient's health or disease, and the strain of cordyceps being tested. The whole matter could probably be cleared up if the same strain of cordyceps were used in a battery of experiments, but so far that research has not been done. Nevertheless, the evidence to date suggests that cordyceps has great potential as an excellent immunoregulator.

CHAPTER 9

CORDYCEPS
AND FATIGUE

A colleague in Los Angeles recently asked me to look into cordyceps as a remedy for fatigue. The doctor had been swamped with patients complaining of symptoms that suggested the outbreak of some new contagious disease. But after undergoing a barrage of tests, it seemed that all the patients were suffering from *chronic fatigue.* She prescribed plenty of rest and suggested that they consider taking some supplements. She then asked me for advice. Except for ginseng, the only other supplement that came to mind was cordyceps, partly because the herbalists of ancient China had recognized its similarities to ginseng. A month or so later, she called back to say that several of her most fatigued patients had tried it, and all claimed to be doing very much better.

My colleague was then consulted by several patients who were unable to recover from *chronic fatigue syndrome* despite having been treated by a number of specialists, including naturopaths, chiropractors, and herbalists. She suggested that they try cordyceps since it had seemed to help her patients with chronic fatigue, a condition with similar symptoms. She told me they had tried it with very positive results. This led me to begin investigating the use of cordyceps in treating chronic fatigue and chronic fatigue syndrome.

WHAT IS FATIGUE?

Fatigue is often misdiagnosed. In fact, fatigue accompanies almost all diseases and is typified by general weakness or malaise. The word comes from the Latin *fatigare,* which means to exhaust or to weary. Fatigue implies mental or physical exhaustion, and is characterized by a temporary reduction in energy following a period of prolonged activity, stimulation, or illness. One article defines fatigue as "a subjective, unpleasant symptom [that] incorporates total body feelings ranging from tiredness to exhaustion, creating an unrelenting overall condition [that] interferes with individuals' ability to function to their normal capacity."[1] Another definition emphasizes the complex nature of fatigue as a "self-recognized state in which an individual experiences an overwhelming sustained sense of exhaustion and decreased capacity for physical and mental work that is not relieved by rest."[2]

One factor that can lead to a state of fatigue is repetitive work, especially after prolonged periods. Researchers at the Human Factors Research Laboratory at the University of Minnesota suggest that when fatigue is caused by repetitive work, the best remedy is rest.

But rest is not a panacea. A pilot study listed factors reported to exacerbate fatigue in patients: age, disease, emotional stress, environmental factors, lack of social support, medications and treatments, nutritional status, overexertion, and sleep quantity and quality. When fatigue is accompanied by lack of sleep over a period of weeks and months, it becomes a chronic medical problem. In the following sections, we will take a look at two forms of fatigue, *chronic fatigue* and *chronic fatigue syndrome,* and how they can be alleviated with cordyceps.

Chronic Fatigue

Chronic forms of fatigue have been found in 25 percent of patients under the care of physicians. Unfortunately, these patients don't readily fit classifications used by the international psychiatric community, and they are often neglected. One study found that patients with severe chronic fatigue were particularly disabled in areas of vitality, social functioning, and the ability to carry out day-to-day activities. The intensity of their disabilities and patterns of dysfunction were significantly different from those of patients with major depression, and their mental health and emotional functioning were fairly preserved.

Researchers at the Chronic Fatigue Clinic of the University of Washington in Seattle reported that 26 percent of the chronic fatigue patients they had surveyed were unemployed. And among the employed chronic fatigue patients, 23 percent reported that their performance at work had decreased. Patients suffering from chronic fatigue have a number of problems in common. Let's take a look at some indications of chronic fatigue.

- Need for long periods of sleep

- Poor sleep

- Poor concentration

- Poor memory

- Speech problems (for example, inability to find the right word)

- Muscle pain following physical activity and during rest

- Headaches

A recent large-scale study in England found that the prevalence of chronic fatigue was 11.3 percent, which appears to be an accurate figure because it corresponds with the 11.2 percent estimated by a previous survey in England. It is generally believed that the percentage of patients who are suffering from chronic fatigue and are under the primary or secondary care of a physician ranges from 10 to as high as 40 percent. One study found that 38 percent of patients seeing a general practitioner for various ailments were in fact suffering from fatigue.

Chronic fatigue patients have a more difficult time coping with their ailment than do nonfatigued patients suffering from other ailments. In addition, they seem to be more physically impaired, endure more pain, and suffer from reduced mental health. Their perception of their health is also less positive. A clearer picture of how much these patients suffer emerged when researchers found that patients with arthritis, hypertension, and diabetes were better able to function than those with chronic fatigue. The only patients whose functioning was more handicapped were those with advanced stage coronary artery disease and angina.

The only beneficial treatment for patients with chronic fatigue is rest. In some cases, antidepressants can help, but there's no proof that they work any better than placebos.

Cordyceps and Chronic Fatigue

My conviction that cordyceps is effective in helping people with chronic fatigue is supported by the case of Father Perennin, whose fatigue and exhaustion were cured by cordyceps. Another indicator is its use by Chinese athletes as a sports supplement, or post-exercise recovery food; and in fact a number of American athletes have begun to take cordyceps for the same reason. These testimonies and the knowledge that cordyceps has long been used by doctors of traditional Chinese medicine in cases of excessive tiredness suggest that it can help people suffering from chronic fatigue.

Chronic Fatigue Syndrome (CFS)

Chronic fatigue syndrome, or CFS, is diagnosed when there is persistent or relapsing chronic fatigue for more than six months that is not the result of overexertion and that is not alleviated by rest. There is also a substantial reduction in levels of personal, educational, social, or occupational activities and the presence of at least four of the following:

- Muscle pain

- Headaches

- Unrefreshing sleep

- Postexertion malaise

- Multijoint pain

- Sore throat

- Tenderness of the axillary lymph nodes or cervical lymph nodes

- Memory impairment or impaired concentration

Although chronic fatigue syndrome is a recognized disease, most physicians have not learned to diagnose it accurately. Consequently, patients often require the services of a specialist for a correct diagnosis. CFS is a controversial subject in Western medicine. This is probably because it has a strong psychological component. Approximately 50 percent of CFS patients suffer from depression and about 25 percent have minor depression, anxiety disorders, and phobia. Another reason for the controversy is that no single test or biological aspect has yet determined the presence of chronic fatigue syndrome. All the same, the controversy over CFS is probably the major reason for a long-overdue renewal of interest in chronic fatigue, and the state of fatigue itself.

If you suspect that you have CFS, it is extremely important to eliminate the possibility that another disease is causing the problem. Low blood pressure and liver diseases are especially known for producing fatigue; and cancer, AIDS, tuberculosis, and depression must not be overlooked. Treatment of CFS is experimental, even in conventional medicine. Nevertheless, many people do recover with alternative treatments. And it is for this reason that we turn our attention to cordyceps.

Cordyceps and CFS

The use of cordyceps by doctors of traditional Chinese medicine to treat excessive tiredness is one of the surest indications that it may be helpful to chronic fatigue syndrome. As our understanding of CFS evolves, perhaps cordyceps will become a more enticing subject for research into this perplexing disease. The pharmacological indications that cordyceps might prove beneficial to patients with CFS are limited by the lack of agreement about the biological and biochemical signs of the disease, a topic sure to remain controversial for years to come.

If cordyceps benefits CFS patients, how does it work? Laboratory findings on cordyceps and CFS reveal some interesting facts. For example, researchers have reported that CFS patients have an unusual form of adrenal insufficiency and, oddly enough, high levels of male hormones. This adrenal insufficiency may help account for the neuropsychological abnormalities and the muscle dysfunction seen in CFS patients. The fact that cordyceps enhances the function of the adrenal cortex is one indication that it may help people suffering from chronic fatigue syndrome. In addition, chronic fatigue syndrome patients often have moderate dysfunction in respiratory muscle performance, which can be helped by cordyceps. CFS patients often experience problems of the *HPA axis*, which involves the pituitary gland and responds to stressful events by producing chemical messengers that bring feelings of despair. And finally, CFS often produces a significant reduction in urinary and plasma levels of *glucocorticoids*—natural hormones produced by the body to protect against stress. Cordyceps can strengthen the resiliency or integrity of the HPA axis and it seems to alleviate stress, thus calming the nervous system.

CONCLUSION

Although there are indications that cordyceps alleviates fatigue, more research must be conducted to prove its effectiveness. However, as you have seen, people suffering from various forms of fatigue who have tried cordyceps already report more than satisfactory results.

CHAPTER 10

GUIDELINES FOR USING CORDYCEPS

You now have an excellent idea of how cordyceps can help in the treatment of a number of disorders. And you have learned that it can enhance your general health when taken as a dietary supplement. But where can you find cordyceps, and how much should you take?

HOW TO SELECT CORDYCEPS

The best quality cordyceps products are standardized to contain a given amount of active constituents in every dose. This way you can be sure of getting the same amount every time, and you can gauge how much to take for your particular needs. Look for labels that state whether the product is standardized, derived from mycelium or wild cordyceps, extracted or ground into a powder. Furthermore, make sure that the label provides the scientific name along with the common name of the product, and the recommended dosage should be clearly indicated. A good company will also include a telephone number, and some offer an e-mail address for further information.

High-quality cordyceps products generally produce

noticeable effects within the first week and more obvious results within three to six weeks. The most convenient products are encapsulated and supplied in a lightproof bottle.

Which Product Should You Choose?

A number of mycelial cordyceps products are now available in U.S. pharmacies and health food stores. Cordyceps is also sold on the Web, although often without sufficient product information to warrant being listed here. Table 10.1 may help you decide which may be the best for you. To learn more about any of the individual products listed below, see the resource list on page 109.

Table 10.1. Cordyceps Products

Brand: *Cordyceps Gold*

Label: *Cordyceps sinensis* cultured mycelium powder; standardized to 10% cordycepic acid (mannitol) and at least 1% cordycepin (indicator of nucleotide and adenosine content).

Comment: None

Brand: *CordyMax Cs-4*

Label: *Cordyceps sinensis*-derived mycelium (derived from *Paecilomyces hepiali*) and fermented on soy bean-based nutrient medium; standardized to contain adenosine and mannitol (indicator of polysaccharide content).

Comment: The Cs-4 strain is the same one tested in numerous studies cited in this book.

Brand: *Cordyceps Mycelium Extract*

Label: Capsules containing *Cephalosporium sinensis* (from *Cordyceps sinensis*); contains polysaccharides, sterols, and adenosine as active constituents; mycelium grown on organic brown rice; liquid extract of *Cordyceps sinensis* mycelium extract; liquid culture of *Cordyceps sinensis* mushrooms; active constituents listed as adenosine, polysaccharides, and sterols.

Comment: Some of the studies on cordyceps mentioned in this book used the strain *Cephalosporium sinensis,* which is derived from *Cordyceps sinensis.*

Wild Cordyceps

Chinese herb stores often carry the wild form of cordyceps. The problem with the wild form is that it may not be free from bacterial contaminants. In fact, wild cordyceps was recently responsible for two cases of lead poisoning in Taiwan. One powdered product contained 414 micrograms of lead per gram, and another was found to contain 20,000 micrograms of lead per gram. The patient had consumed over 2 grams of lead by the time doctors treated her. Health authorities determined that tiny lead bars had been inserted into the freshly picked fungus before drying to increase the weight of the harvest and the resulting profits. Although merchants in the United States are aware of this practice and watch for contamination, there is always the chance that some contaminated cordyceps will get through. The other main problem with the wild form is that it is rarely, if ever, standardized to guarantee potency from one batch to the next.

With these warnings in mind, you may still prefer to use wild cordyceps. You can prepare it in a number of ways. In traditional Chinese medicine, cordyceps is prepared as an herbal tea by adding 3 to 9 grams of wild cordyceps to boiling water and allowing it to simmer for about forty-five minutes. The liquid is then strained and allowed to cool before drinking the tea twice daily. This method is used to prepare cordyceps for the treatment of anemia, coughs, sexual impotence, excessive tiredness, and night sweats. It is also a mild sedative, or calming beverage, which is recommended for increasing stamina, especially during convalescence from an illness. As a general tonic, cordyceps is eaten with chicken, in which case both are steamed together in a pressure cooker. The same preparation is made with pork and taken for impotence or anemia.

Cordyceps is sometimes marinated for ten days in sorghum wine, which is made from a kind of grass used as a source of grain, forage, and sugar. The recipe is said to be good for lower back pain and other pains around the waist area and knees. Would another kind of wine work just as well? Very likely. However, you may be able to find sorghum wine in Chinese foods stores in the United States.

Dosages and Indications

How can you determine the best dosage of cordyceps for you? Table 10.2 provides general guidelines and suggestions for treating specific disorders, as well as for the maintenance of good health. Please note that these suggestions—which include a suggested form of cordyceps—are based on the results of scientific studies. To learn which products are likely to contain the indicated form,

Table 10.2. Dosages and Indications

Indication	Dosage	Product and Form
Acute pulmonary heart disease	1 gram 3 times daily	Cs-4 cultured mycelium powder
Arrhythmias	1,500 mg daily	Cs-4 cultured mycelium powder
Cancer symptoms	1–2 grams 3 times daily	Cs-4 cultured mycelium powder
Cancer therapy side effects	2–3 grams daily	Cs-4 cultured mycelium powder
Chronic bronchitis	1 gram 3 times daily	Cs-4 cultured mycelium powder

Indication	Dosage	Product and Form
Chronic kidney failure	3–6 grams daily	Cs-4 cultured mycelium powder
Chronic obstructive pulmonary disease (COPD)	1 gram 3 times daily	Cs-4 cultured mycelium powder
General weakness	1 gram 3 times daily	Cs-4 cultured mycelium powder
Health maintenance	2 grams daily	*Cordyceps sinensis,* wild or mycelial
Hepatitis B	1.5 grams daily	*Cephalosporium sinensis* mycelium
High blood viscosity	1 gram 3 times daily	Cs-4 cultured mycelium powder
High cholesterol levels	1 gram 3 times daily	Cs-4 cultured mycelium powder
High lipoperoxide levels	1 gram 3 times daily	Cs-4 cultured mycelium powder
Increased SOD levels	1 gram 3 times daily	Cs-4 cultured mycelium powder
Kidneys—to protect against antibiotics	4.5 grams daily	Cs-4 cultured mycelium powder
Kidney—to protect against cyclosporine	1 gram 3 times daily	Cs-4 cultured mycelium powder
Male erectile dysfunction	1 gram 3 times daily	Cs-4 cultured mycelium powder
Posthepatitis cirrhosis	6 to 9 grams daily	Cultivated mycelium product
Quality of life in chronic heart failure	3–4 grams daily	Cs-4 cultured mycelium powder

How Is Cordyceps Classified?

There are many different types of cordyceps. The wild cordy-ceps found in the mountains of Tibet and China is now pro-duced in the laboratory, and it is not always easy to deter-mine what the differences are among the various strains. To make matters worse, the names of the cultured strains are not always included on the label; but to be correct they should appear somewhere. Among the bewildering array of names of derivative cultured species that we might expect to see in mycelial products are **Cephalosporium sinensis, Paecilomyces sinensis, Scytalidium hepiali, Hirsutella sinensis,** *and* **Mortierella hepiali.** *Allow me to explain the use of these names, which are confusing to nearly everyone, including many a mushroom scientist, or mycologist.*

*Mycologists who classify mushrooms have found that many species reproduce without reaching a sexual stage. When this is the case, they are called imperfect fungi (**fungi imperfecti**) to distinguish them from mushrooms that do reproduce from a sexual stage. Because their life cycle lacks*

please see Table 10.1 presented earlier in the chapter. Of course, if you are already taking medication, be sure to consult with your doctor before taking any supplement, including cordyceps.

ISSUES OF SAFETY

As we have stated a number of times, cordyceps is nontox-ic, and there is generally no danger of overdosing on this medicinal herb. The only precaution I can suggest is to be careful when using cordyceps for diseases attended with bleeding. Because cordyceps contains adenosine and relat-

a sexual, or perfect, stage, they represent a point of evolution in the lifecycle of otherwise perfect fungi. As a result, they don't meet the usual classification system requirements used in naming mushrooms.

*The physical characteristics of the mushroom are different in their imperfect form, so mycologists use a different set of names to classify them. The mushrooms may be derived and grown from a culture taken from the same mushroom, they may have the same constituents in the same amounts found in the wild form, and they may even produce the same medicinal activities in clinical and laboratory studies. This is the case with **Paecilomyces hepiali,** or Cs-4, which was separated from **Cordyceps sinensis.** Therefore, a much simpler way of distinguishing the imperfect fungus is to call it **Cordyceps sinensis** Cs-4.*

*Is one strain of cordyceps better than another? The imperfect fungus **Paecilomyces hepiali** seems to be most like the wild cordyceps used by the ancient Chinese herbalists. It is also the strain that has been given the most attention by scientists.*

ed nucleosides, this precaution makes sense because mushrooms rich in these compounds are known to thin the blood. Although, as you know, this has therapeutic value when dealing with atherosclerosis and high blood viscosity, cordyceps could have an additive effect if patients are already taking blood-thinning medications such as aspirin or warfarin. If you are on such medications and you want to take cordyceps, make sure that you are closely monitored by a doctor.

Cordyceps has not yet been adequately evaluated for use by children and pregnant or lactating women. Therefore, it is advisable that medical authorization is given before these people use cordyceps.

The only reports of side effects from cordyceps in clinical studies were mild upper gastrointestinal tract discomfort, nausea, and dry mouth in some patients. These side effects were rare. In addition, there was one case in which a patient developed an allergic reaction to Cs-4. Nevertheless, among clinicians who have studied patients taking Cs-4, the consensus of opinion is that this strain is very safe.

CONCLUSION

Although cordyceps is an extremely safe supplement that can be beneficial to most people, it is recommended that you follow the guidelines in this chapter for dosage and product type. And remember that with cordyceps, as with all herbal medicines, you must be patient and persistent. Don't expect to see results for at least a month or two, or sometimes three. However, the payoff comes without the kinds of risks associated with many prescription drugs.

CONCLUSION

For the first time, people living in Western nations are considering the use of alternative medical treatments. We in the West are now looking to China and other societies for their wealth of knowledge about traditional approaches to healing—approaches ranging from acupuncture to the use of herbs. And Western scientists are proving that many of these treatments do indeed work.

This book was written to provide information about cordyceps so that you, too, can benefit from its unique properties. As a general health supplement, cordyceps increases vitality and a feeling of well-being, especially in people over fifty. It raises levels of the so-called good cholesterol, or HDL form, and reduces levels of lipoperoxide, which can lead to atherosclerosis. Cordyceps has also been shown to help protect various organs of the body such as the liver, the heart, the kidneys, and the lungs. Furthermore, compared with many prescription medications, cordyceps is nontoxic, safe, and convenient to take.

I have seen many success stories in my own patients who have used cordyceps. And my enthusiasm for the herb is bolstered by the results of research conducted by Chinese and Western doctors. I have no hesitation in recommending cordyceps to you if you wish to try it, provided that you let your personal physician know of your intent. Your doctor may be able to help you monitor the results and advise you according to your medical needs. Indeed, there are increasing numbers of Western doctors who are becoming sufficiently knowledgeable about herbal medicines such as cordyceps, and they are beginning to prescribe them to their patients.

Remember that in using any treatments with which you are unfamiliar, it is important to find and work with a healthcare professional who is knowledgeable about alternative treatments. It is vital, too, to stay informed about the latest findings in the field of health through literature written by experts in their fields. It is hoped that this book will be a first step toward greater health and vitality through natural remedies.

ENDNOTES

CHAPTER 1

1. C.G. Lloyd, *"Cordyceps sinesis,"* *Mycological Notes* 54 (1918): 766.

2. Y.C. Wang, "Mycology in Ancient China with Emphasis on Review of the Ancient Literature," *Acta Mycologica Sinica* 4, No. 3 (1995): 133.

3. J. Pereira, "Summer-Plant-Winter-Worm," *New York Journal of Medicine* 1 (1843): 128.

CHAPTER 6

1. M.S. Markell, "Herbal Therapies and the Patient with Kidney Disease," *Quarterly Review of Natural Medicine* (Fall 1997): 189.

CHAPTER 9

1. P.A. Hancock and W.B. Verwey, "Workload and Adaptive Driver Systems," *Accident Analysis and Prevention* 29, No. 4 (1997): 495.

2. L.J. Carpenito, *Nursing Diagnosis: Application to Clinical Practice,* 5th edition. (Philadelphia: J.B. Lippincott, 1995), 26.

SELECTED REFERENCES

Barnes, P.J. "COPD: New Opportunities for Drug Development." *Trends in Pharmacological Sciences* 19, No. 10 (1998): 415–423.

Beinfield, H., and E. Korngold. "Chinese Traditional Medicine: An Introductory Overview." *Alternative Therapies* 1, No. 1 (1995): 44–52.

Bennet, J.C., and F. Plum, eds. *Cecil Textbook of Medicine.* Philadelphia: W.B. Saunders, 1996.

Buchwald, D., T. Pearlman, J. Umali, et al. "Functional Status in Patients with Chronic Fatigue Syndrome, Other Fatiguing Illnesses, and Healthy Individuals." *The American Journal of Medicine* 101, No. 4 (1996): 364–370.

Carpenito, L.J. *Nursing Diagnosis: Application to Clinical Practice.* Philadelphia: J.B. Lippincott, 1995.

Chang, H.M., and P.H Butt, eds. *Pharmacology and Applications of Chinese Materia Medica* 1. Philadelphia: World Scientific, 1986.

Che, Y.S., and L.Z. Lin "Observation on Therapeutic Effects of JinShuiBao on Coronary Heart Disease, Hyperlipidemia, and Blood Rheology." *Chinese Traditional and Herbal Drugs* 27, No. 9 (1996): 552–553.

Chen, D.G. "Effects of JinShuiBao Capsule on the Quality of Life of Patients with Heart Failure." *Journal of Administration of Traditional Chinese Medicine* 5 (1995): 40–43.

Clark, A.L. and T. McDonough. "The Origin of Symptoms in Chronic Heart Failure." *Heart* 78, No. 5 (1995): 429–430.

Crouse, S.F., B.C. O'Brian, P.W. Grandjean, et al. "Effects of Training and a Single Session of Exercise on Lipids and Apolipoproteins in Hypercholesterolemic Men." *Journal of Applied Physiology* 83, No. 6 (1997): 2,019–2,028.

Donohue, J.F. "Recent Advances in the Treatment of Asthma." *Current Opinion in Pulmonary Medicine* 2 (1996): 1–6.

Du Halde, P. *The General History of China.* London: John Watts, 1736.

Fukuda, K., S.E. Straus, I. Hicki, et al. "Chronic Fatigue Syndrome: A Comprehensive Approach to its Definition and Study." *Annals of Internal Medicine* 121 (1994): 953–959.

Guo, Y.Z. "Medicinal Chemistry, Pharmacology, and Clinical Applications of Fermented Mycelia of *Cordyceps sinensis* and JinShuiBao Capsule." *Journal of Modern Diagnostics and Therapeutics* 1 (1986): 60–65.

Hancock, P.A., and W.B. Verwey. "Fatigue, Workload and Adaptive Driver Systems." *Accident Analysis and Prevention* 29, No. 4 (1997): 495–506.

Huang, Y.M., J.B. Lu, B.C. Zhu, et al. "Toxicity Study of Fermentation Cordyceps B414." *Zhongchengyao Yanjiu* 10 (1987): 24–25.

Jiang, J.C., and Y.F. Cao. "Summary of Treatment of 37 Chronic Renal Dysfunction Patients with JinShuiBao." *Journal of Administration of Traditional Chinese Medicine* 5 (1995): 23–24.

Juvonen, J., T. Juvonen, and P. Saikku. "Can Degenerative Aortic Valve Stenosis Be Related to Persistent *Chlamydia pneumoniae* Infection?" *Annals of Internal Medicine* 128, No. 9 (1998): 741.

Kashyap, M.L. "Cholesterol and Atherosclerosis: A Contemporary Perspective." *Annals Academy of Medicine Singapore* 26, No. 4 (1997): 517–523.

Kennedy, H.L. "Beta Blockade, Ventricular Arrhythmias, and Sudden Cardiac Death." *American Journal of Cardiology* 80, No. 9B (1997): 29J-34J.

Keys, John D. *Chinese Herbs: Their Botany, Chemistry, and Pharmacodynamics.* Rutland, VT: Charles E. Tuttle Company, 1976.

Kubzansky, L.D., I. Kawachi, A. Spiro, et al. "Is Worrying Bad for Your Heart?" *Circulation* 95 (1997): 818–824.

Lei, M. and J.P. Wang "JinShuiBao Capsule as Adjuvant Treatment for Acute Stage Pulmonary Heart Disease: Analysis of Therapeutic Effect of 50 Clinical Cases." *Journal of Administration of Traditional Chinese Medicine* 5 (1995): 28–29.

Lemanske, R.F. "Asthma." *Journal of the American Medical Association* 278 (1997): 1855–1873.

Lin, Anna. *A Handbook of TCM Urology and Male Sexual Dysfunction.* Boulder, CO: Blue Poppy Press, Inc., 1992.

Liu, B. and Y.S, Bau. *Fungi Pharmacopoeia* (Sinica). Oakland, CA: The Kinoko Company, 1980.

Liu, C., H.M. Xue, L.M. Xu, et al. "Treatment of 22 Patients with Post-Hepatitis Cirrhosis with a Preparation of Fermented Mycelia of *Cordyceps sinensis.*" *Shanghai Journal of Chinese Materia Medica* 6 (1986): 30–31.

Lloyd, C.G. "*Cordyceps sinensis.*" *Mycological Notes* 54 (1918): 766–76.

Manfreds, D. et al. "Morbidity and Mortality from Chronic Obstructive Pulmonary Disease." *Annual Review of Respiratory Disease* 140 (1992): S19–S26.

Markell, M.S. "Herbal Therapies and the Patient with Kidney Disease." *Quarterly Review of Natural Medicine* (Fall 1997): 189–200.

McGuffin, M., et al. *Botanical Safety Handbook.* Boca Raton, FL: CRC Press, 1997.

Mizuno, T., T. Sakai, and G. Chihara. "Health Foods and Medicinal Usage of Mushrooms." *Food Reviews International* 11, No. 1 (1995): 69–81.

Pegler, D.N., Y.J. Yao, and Y. Li. "The Chinese Caterpillar Fungus." *The Mycologist* 8 (1994): 3–5.

Pereira, J. "Summer-Plant-Winter-Worm." *New York Journal of Medicine* 1 (1843): 128–132.

Shao, G., Z.H. You, Y.C. Cu, et al. "Treatment of Hyperlipidemia with *Cordyceps sinensis:* A Double-Blind Placebo-Control Trial." *International Journal of Oriental Medicine* 15, No. 2 (1990): 77–80.

Steinkraus, D.C., and J.B. Whitfield. "Chinese Caterpillar Fungus and World Record Runners." *American Entomologist* (Winter 1994): 235–239.

Uoma, P.V.I., S. Nayha, K. Sikkila, et. al. "High Serum Alpha-Tocopherol, Albumin, Selenium and Cholesterol, and Low Mortality from Coronary Heart Disease in Northern Finland." *Journal of Internal Medicine* 237 (1995): 49–54.

Wan, F., Y. Guo, and X. Deng. "Sex Hormone-Like Effects of JinShuiBao Capsule: Pharmacological and Clinical Studies." *Chinese Traditional Patent Medicine* 9 (1988): 29–31.

Wang, Q., and Y. Zhao. "Comparison of Some Pharmacological Effects Between *Cordyceps sinesis* and *Cephalosporium sinesis.*" *Bulletin of Chinese Materia Medica* 12 (1987): 682–684.

Wang, Y.C. "Mycology in Ancient China With Emphasis on Review of the Ancient Literature." *Acta Mycologica Sinica* 4, No. 3 (1995): 133–140.

Watkins, W. "Mind-Body Pathways." *Mind-Body Medicine: A Clinicians Guide to Psychoneuroimmunology.* New York: Churchill Livingstone (1997): 1–15.

Yamaguchi, N., J. Yoshida, L.J. Ren, et al. "Augmentation of Various Immune Reactivities of Tumor-Bearing Hosts with an Extract of *Cordyceps sinensis.*" *Biotherapy* 2, No. 3 (1990): 199–205.

Xie, F.Y. "Therapeutic Observation of Xingbao in Treating 83 Patients with Asymptomatic Hepatitis B." *Chinese Journal of Hospital Pharmacy* 12, No. 8 (1992): 352–353.

Xu, J.M., and H.J. Zheng. "Treating 64 Patients with Arrhythmia by Ningxinbao Capsule: A Randomized, Double-Blind Observation." *Shanghai Journal of Traditional Chinese Medicine* 4 (1994): 4–5.

Yen, K.Y. *The Illustrated Chinese Materia Medica: Crude and Prepared.* Taipei, Taiwan: SMC Publishing, Inc., 1992.

Yue, D., et al. *Advanced Study for Traditional Chinese Herbal Medicine. Institute of Materia Medica.* Beijing: Beijing Medical University and China Peking Union Medical University Press, 1995.

Zhang, M., and N. Kinjo. "Notes on the Alpine Cordyceps of China and Nearby Nations." *Mycotaxon* 66 (1998): 215–229.

Zhang, Z., W. Huang, S. Liao, et al. "Clinical and Laboratory Studies of JinShuiBao in Scavenging Oxygen Free Radicals in Elderly Senescent XuZheng Patients." *Journal of Administration of Traditional Chinese Medicine* 5 (1995): 14–18.

Zhou, D.H., and L.Z. Lin. "Effect of Jinshuibao Capsule on the Immunological Function of 36 Patients with Advanced Cancer." *Chung Kuo Chung Hsi I Chieh Ho Tsa Chih* 15, No. 8 (1995): 476–478.

Zhu, J.S., G.M. Halpern, and K. Jones. "The Scientific Rediscovery of an Ancient Chinese Herbal Medicine: *Cordyceps sinesis.* Part I." *Journal of Alternative and Contemporary Medicine* 4, No. 3 (1998): 289–303.

RESOURCE LIST

Cordyceps products can be found in many pharmacies, Chinese herb stores, health-food stores, and on the World Wide Web. But if you have difficulty finding what you're looking for, the following list should guide you to a manufacturer or supplier who can either sell the desired product to you directly or inform you of the nearest retail outlet.

Fungi Perfecti
P.O. Box 7634
Olympia, WA 98507
(800) 780-9126
www.fungi.com

Garuda International, Inc.
P.O. Box 5155
Santa Cruz, CA 95063
(831) 462-6341
www.garudaint.com

North American Reishi, Ltd.
P.O. Box 1780
Gibsons, BC V0N 1V0
Canada
(604) 886-7799
reishi@sunshine.net

Pharmanex, Inc.
One Nu Skin Plaza
75 West Center Street
Provo, UT 84601
(800) 800-0260
www.pharmanex.com

Resources

Index